MW01000352

Braver Than You Think

BRAVER
THAN
YOU
THINK

———⊷⊶———

Around the World on the Trip
of My (Mother's) Lifetime

MAGGIE DOWNS

COUNTERPOINT
Berkeley, California

BRAVER THAN YOU THINK

Braver Than You Think is a work of nonfiction. Events have been reconstructed from
notes, blog posts, personal journal entries, and my own subjective memory. Some
names and other identifying characteristics have been changed to protect privacy. In
some instances, I compressed time, removed people, and skipped over locations. (For
the latter, I apologize to the entire country of Laos. I was very happy there.)

Library of Congress Cataloging-in-Publication Data
Names: Downs, Maggie, author.
Title: Braver than you think : around the world on the trip of my (mother's) lifetime /
    Maggie Downs.
Description: First hardcover edition. | Berkeley, California : Counterpoint, 2020.
Identifiers: LCCN 2019030639 | ISBN 9781640092921 (hardcover) | ISBN
    9781640092938 (ebook)
Subjects: LCSH: Downs, Maggie—Travel. | Downs, Maggie—Family. | Voyages
    around the world. | Backpacking. | Alzheimer's disease—Patients—Family
    relationships. | Terminally ill parents—United States. | Mothers and daughters—
    United States. | Parent and adult child—United States. | Women authors—
    Biography. | Authors, American—21st century—Biography.
Classification: LCC G440.D74 A3 2020 Y DDC 910.4/1092 [B]—dc23
LC record available at https://lccn.loc.gov/2019030639

Jacket design by Sarah Brody
Book design by Jordan Koluch

COUNTERPOINT
2560 Ninth Street, Suite 318
Berkeley, CA 94710
www.counterpointpress.com

Printed in the United States of America
Distributed by Publishers Group West

10 9 8 7 6 5 4 3 2 1

For Mutti. You were with me even when you weren't.

No one expected me. Everything awaited me.

—PATTI SMITH

Contents

Braver Than You Think

Prologue

⊶⊶⊷

THE AIRPLANE BEGINS ITS DESCENT INTO CAIRO, BUT I don't even look out the window. I've had the shade drawn the whole twelve hours, all the way from the United States, a time in which I didn't sleep but was not awake either.

Sorrow does that.

I shuffle off the plane in what has become my standard uniform: navy flip-flops and hiking pants that unzip just above the knee to convert into shorts. The hood of my sweatshirt is pulled over my head, my long, unruly curls tucked inside the fabric. If anyone bothered to look at me, they'd see red, gutted eyes and a clenched jaw, not the kind of person they'd want to make conversation with anyway.

The last time I landed in Cairo, it was a different story. I had a window seat then too, and I didn't close the shade at all. I pressed my face to the smudgy plastic, watched the green band of Nile slice through the billowy, beige fabric of the country. As the aircraft descended, the land appeared to breathe—the mountains, the dunes, the shifting sands. It was like a golden exhale. Even closer to the ground, the light of the city shifted with glass and metal, glowing like a tiger's-eye stone. My cheeks flushed with warmth; my eyes felt clear and open. I chattered with strangers at baggage claim. I made conversation with the taxi driver.

That was almost a month ago. Before my mother died of Alzheimer's disease. Before I traveled home to Ohio for a funeral, buried my mom on a snowy day, and flew back to a desert, shrouded in grief and fleece. Before.

But now something else is off, too. At the airport I try calling home from one of the pay phones, just to let my family know that I made it to my destination, but the line is dead. I try each phone. None of them work.

The airport internet café is closed. When I ask how I can get online or make a call, I am met with shrugs. That's when I notice the men in uniforms, standing in the airport windows.

My eyes are wild now, scanning the crowd. There are businesspeople in suits, women in head scarves, men in galabias that drag along the ground. Children and teenagers, suitcases and strollers. Nobody else seems panicked. But now I pick out soldiers, armed and walking among the travelers. They carry themselves with the unmistakable air of authority, their footfalls purposeful and strong. Though the security is impressively tight at the Cairo airport, I don't remember such a strong military presence before.

My eye finally lands on a TV, where a crowd is gathering to watch BBC News. The footage shows tanks and rioters, piles of people throwing stones and wrestling each other to the ground. The background of the footage begins to take shape and look familiar. It's Tahrir Square, just a block from the hostel where I intended to stay.

A red graphic with bold letters flashes across the screen: "Egypt in crisis!" My face blooms hot and red. My eyes water. A tremor quakes through my entire body, and I force myself to remain standing. It is January 25, 2011, the day of rage, the day the Arab Spring ignites.

My mom is dead. I am alone, far from home. And a revolution has begun.

LOVE

—⊸∞⊶—

Has it ever struck you that life is all memory, except for the one present moment that goes by you so quick you hardly catch it going?

—TENNESSEE WILLIAMS

You Are Braver Than You Think

—⸺∞⸺—

Jason wraps his lean body around me and squeezes me tightly. It is July 8, 2010, the first night of our honeymoon. Some might mistake our embrace for passion, but mostly we are just cold on the floor of the Lima international airport, huddled together for warmth.

"Great honeymoon, sweetie," Jason says through clenched teeth. His dark hair is rumpled, and his jawline is rough with stubble. Black-framed glasses sit askew on his face, one side of which rests against a sweatshirt turned pillow.

He's joking. But I do wonder how great this honeymoon will be, knowing we're about to split up.

Technically this trip to Peru is our first romantic getaway as a married couple. But it is also the launch of my yearlong trip around the world, an idea that took root as my mother entered the final stages of Alzheimer's disease.

I hatched the plan in 2009, ten years into my career in daily newspapers. Ten years of work and accolades—my desk was a mountain of notebooks and files, along with plaques for best reporter, best features writer, best column writing of the company—but ten years of telling other people's stories, not my own.

Even though the job brought me to Palm Springs, California, where I met interesting people, it felt like my world had telescoped into something small, insignificant. I couldn't envision much beyond the nubby carpet walls of my newsroom cubicle. And travel? I barely made enough to cover rent in Southern California. How far could I get during my allotted two weeks of vacation?

So the idea seemed wild at first: what if I quit my job and spent a year traveling the world to complete the journey my mother never had a chance to make?

But as it began to marinate, the idea seemed less than wild. It felt necessary. My mom had a lot of goals, and she put them off to raise a family. To raise my sister, my brother, and me. Then she was diagnosed with Alzheimer's in 2001, before she ever accomplished any of the things she wanted to do. By confining my life to my cubicle, wasn't I making the same mistake my mother made? Why was I lingering when I could be living—the very thing my mom wanted most?

Three yard sales, several plane reservations, and one resignation letter later, here I am.

Even though my mom never created a formal bucket list, I've brainstormed nine things around the world that she wanted to do but didn't. The plan is for Jason to spend three weeks with me in Peru, then return to California. After he is gone, I will continue on my own through South America, then Africa and Asia, checking things off my list for Mom and achieving a few of my personal goals too.

I've never heard of anyone else leaving a marriage like this. Not on purpose, while it is still new and good and fresh. I am grateful Jason loves me enough to let me leave, but I know it's a risk. This year of monogamous separation will either make us stronger or wrench us apart for good. It will prove that I can make one revolution of the planet and find my way home again.

Or that I can't.

This part about sleeping at the airport was my idea to maximize time and money. We had been in motion all day long, driving from my friend's house in Moreno Valley to the Los Angeles airport, then flying to Panama City, and then to Lima. Our flight arrived past midnight, and our next flight—a quick, one-hour hop to Cusco, Peru—is scheduled to board at 4 a.m. Since there are few budget accommodations within forty miles of the Lima airport, it only made sense to sleep in the airport for a few hours.

"So when I vowed to be with you for better or worse … ?" Jason says.

"Yeah, this is the 'worse' part."

Our sleeping situation appears to be common at this airport, where many international flights arrive late and the domestic flights begin early. The floor smells septic and is littered with the bodies of fallen travelers. The tired and weary are flopped across every possible surface, from the nicotine-stained couches in the smoking lounge to the air-conditioned corners of the food court. My attempt to find a quiet hallway was foiled by a few dozen snoring missionaries in matching red T-shirts.

Jason and I finally found a spot on the floor near the glass wall of an internet café, a place remote enough to not have heavy airport traffic but not remote enough to put us at risk for a mugging.

It turns out crashing on the floor of an airport is one of those things that seems reasonable enough until you actually do it. It's not so great when your cheek is pressed against the tile, watching tumbleweeds of hair and trash roll toward your face.

The floor is as frigid and hard as a slab at the morgue. As people walk past with rolling luggage, I can feel their footsteps in my bones. Every time my eyes close, a scratchy voice comes over the PA system to announce the next international flight or beckon tardy travelers.

Jason and I attempt to sleep, but between us, we have just one sleeping bag. (He planned to rent a sleeping bag in Cusco, so he didn't bother to bring one along.) We unzip my one-person bag and curl together underneath it. I am also clinging to my fifty-pound blue backpack, filled with all my clothes, supplies, and gear for the next year. I am literally sandwiched between everything I love and everything I need.

"You know, other couples stay in four-star hotels for their honeymoons,"

Jason says. But we aren't like other couples, something I knew from the day we met.

FIRST I SHOULD TELL YOU ABOUT THE DISEASE, BECAUSE that's what set everything in motion.

In the year 2000, I was working my first newspaper job out of college, living in Zanesville, a scruffy river town in Southeast Ohio, about two hours away from where my mom and dad lived in a suburb of Dayton. I returned home on the weekends for laundry and meatloaf, frequently enough to notice when my mom stopped wearing her trademark Revlon poppysilk red lipstick. She stopped cooking meals that resembled food. She was scattered and anxious. There was a neighbor's red truck parked down the street, and Mom was convinced someone was spying on her.

Then came the diagnosis that changed everything in her world and in mine. My vibrant, sixty-year-old mom's life began to look like a scrapbook lived in reverse—fragments of memories and snapshots of people plucked away, the stretch of blank pages growing longer, more stark, empty.

Over the next couple of years, my mom had a rapid acceleration of Alzheimer's symptoms. The more she forgot, the more I wanted to gather memories while I still could, to make my time count, to fill the pages of my life. I made lists of what I wanted to accomplish, and I furiously tried to tick off all the to-dos. I moved to a city, got a job as a columnist and reporter for the *Cincinnati Enquirer*, bought wine that came in bottles instead of boxes.

Wait. Scratch that, because that makes it sound like I was doing something nobler than I actually was, which was avoiding the reality of my mom's disease. I did whatever I could to dull the stupid, achy, hot hurt inside, a restless pain that was almost too unbearable to carry. I couldn't face losing my mom piece by piece, so for the most part, I didn't face it.

Even though Cincinnati was just an hour away from my parents, I stopped visiting home unless it was necessary. I went out most nights and knew where to go for the after-parties *after* the after-parties. I dated people, but the wrong ones. And though I often felt bad, I relished feeling something.

That is the context for what happened next: one morning I drove from Cincinnati to an airport hangar in rural Indiana and plunked down the money for my first skydive. I was scared, and I didn't know what to do with my fear except hold it in my body and let it guide me out of an airplane.

There are studies that suggest Alzheimer's is inherited through the mother, and that terrified me far more than any skydive. The woman I loved most in this world, the woman who adored me more than anything in the world, might have already handed off the genetic mutation that will someday kill me.

Who knows how long my own mind will last? I figured. *Why not jump?*

My skydive was an accelerated free fall (or AFF) jump, which meant two instructors would exit the aircraft with me, one on each side of my body. They act as human training wheels, hanging on to my jumpsuit to offer stability and keep me from cartwheeling across the sky. Then, at 5,000 feet, I was supposed to deploy my own parachute and pilot it to the ground. The entirety of this routine, from exit to landing, was practiced during six hours of ground school, which is mandatory before an AFF skydive.

For my jump, I requested that I be paired with anyone but "That Guy"—a shaggy-haired skydiver, ropy and energetic, who looked fresh off the set of a Mountain Dew commercial. He wore mirrored sunglasses, a grass-stained jumpsuit, and a dented helmet, which didn't inspire confidence in his skydiving abilities. He didn't say much, only shouted "Woo!"

"That Guy looks crazy," I said. As I gestured to him, That Guy made eye contact. He stuck out his tongue, winked, and made the hand gesture for "Hang loose!" I disliked him immediately.

When the load manifested, I was assigned my two instructors—Bud, a compact, no-nonsense teacher, and That Guy, whose real name was Jason. My stomach lurched, knowing I was in the hands of this walking, talking sugar high. I didn't want to go anywhere with him, least of all tumbling through the sky at 120 miles per hour.

Jason high-fived me. I pulled my hand away quickly, crossing my arms in front of my chest.

"Are you ready?" It was a question, but it came out like a pep-squad cheer.

"I'm fine," I said. "I'm ready to jump out of a perfectly good airplane."

"Well, the plane's not that good." He smiled.

Jason told the truth. There are no seats inside a skydiving aircraft. Seats waste space and add weight, plus pose a safety risk with all the handles and cords that hang from the rigs. So about fifteen of us sardined together on the floor, leaning against each other with legs splayed. I was positioned in Jason's lap, his arms around me. Bud sat on my feet, which quickly grew numb. I looked around and saw the interior of the plane had been gutted, revealing patches of rust and exposed wires.

It was so cold on the way to altitude that my fingers stiffened and my lips trembled. After practicing a round of hand signals, Jason leaned forward and whispered in my ear.

"Are you okay?" he said.

"Fine."

"Your face is gray," he said.

"I'm fine," I snapped. "My face always looks that way."

At 13,000 feet we were at jump run, when the plane slows for jumpers to exit. One of the skydivers opened the door and leaned his head into the sky. He caught the wind in his mouth, lips flaring to expose his teeth and gums, something out of a horror movie. When he parted his teeth, his fat tongue thwacked against his cheek.

The air that rushed into the plane sucked my breath away. My eyes widened, dry with panic.

"Hey, this is your skydive," Jason said softly. "It's all about what makes you comfortable. If you don't want to do this . . ."

"I do."

The experienced skydivers sang, joyfully launching into the Johnny Cash classic "Ring of Fire." Each time they sang the word "down," my heart lurched a little more. Nervous, I leaned back on Jason for support. I trembled in his arms. He remained steady.

"Hey, if you don't want to jump, I'll ride the plane down with you," he said. "You don't have to do this. Either way, it's okay. Just relax."

He held his right arm in front of my face and made the skydiving hand signal for "relax." It was a loose shaking motion, as if he'd just washed his hands and couldn't find a paper towel.

The plane circled the drop zone, where overlapping runways carved a large, definitive X into the landscape. One by one, the other jumpers waddled to the plane's Narnia door and abruptly vanished, spirited away into another world. The suddenness and completeness of each disappearance made me gasp out loud. They were there. And then they were gone. Irretrievably gone.

I thought about my mom and how she would never see the world from a plane window again. All the goals we chattered about, all the plans we made during late-night conversations, would forever be left unaccomplished, her dreams of travel unreached. She would die, certainly, though a significant part of her was already gone.

For as long as I can remember, my family had a subscription to *National Geographic* magazine, every issue kept on a bookshelf that took up almost one whole wall. Just row after row of mustard-yellow spines. Every month, when a new issue arrived, my mom and I sat at the kitchen table and let the words and images transport us all over the world, from the pyramids in Egypt to the ruins of Machu Picchu, on safari, atop mountains, inside golden temples, through the pink canyons of Petra. These exotic-to-us places could not have been more unreachable from our modest home in Ohio, but there was a kind of magic when Mom and I hatched plans for the future together. They almost seemed possible.

Then my mom took this mental list of adventures and carefully tucked it away, setting her own desires aside to care for our family.

"Someday," she said. "There'll be plenty of time later."

But she was wrong. My mom crept toward death, not one passport stamp closer to her dreams. The woman she wanted to be was just as irretrievable as the skydivers who whooshed out the door.

I looked over my shoulder at Jason and shouted to be heard over the rushing wind.

"I don't know about this," I screamed. And even though I wasn't sure if he could hear me, I continued, "This isn't me. I kind of like the road that is *more* traveled, you know? I'm a beaten-path kind of person."

"Where you're going, there is no path!" he replied with a wink.

The plane was almost empty. Only the pilot and my group remained. Bud crouched in the exit position at the door, just like we rehearsed. He motioned to me.

"You have to make a choice," Jason said. "Now."

He was right. This was my choice. Maybe I wasn't born to be the kind of audacious woman who soaks her weekends in adrenaline. But maybe, just for a little while, I could *choose* to be. There was an urgency that underscored every moment, knowing life—and the disease—might eventually leave me with no choice at all.

I lined my feet up with the edge of the door, right foot in front of the left, and took my position in a half squat, right hand pressed on the inside of the plane, left hand on the outside. The routine I practiced took over my body.

"Check in," I said, and I made eye contact with Bud.

"Check out," I said, and I looked to my left, where Jason hung from the outside of the Caravan with one hand.

"Prop," I said, and I stared ahead at the spinning propeller with laserbeam focus. The vibration of the airplane thrummed in my stomach. The propeller appeared to slow down.

On a count of "up, down, arch," we were out. My spine stiffened and my mind zeroed in on all the wrong things. My shoelace came untied—the plastic tabs on the laces slapped against my ankle—and I wondered if my shoe would get sucked off my foot. Even worse, what if I hit a bird while I was in free fall? My goggles cut into my face. The ground seemed big, a green maw waiting to swallow me whole.

Then I looked to my left, where Jason held my harness, helping me fall sure and true. He cut a handsome figure, hovering there in the pale blue sky, steady by my side. He thrust his hand in front of my face and shook it.

"Relax," he mouthed. And I did. I exhaled. I could do this.

During free fall I had to demonstrate what's called "a circle of awareness"—assess my heading, look to the altimeter on my wrist and call out my altitude, make eye contact with each instructor, and fake deploy three times in a row before the final wave-off.

At 5,000 feet I deployed the parachute for real, and then I drifted gently in the pastel blue expanse. After the speed of free fall, being under canopy felt like drifting through glue. Around me, clouds looked like giant hand-fuls of puffed dough. The air smelled thin, clean, iridescent. Below my feet, the emerald Indiana farmland was studded with houses that almost looked jeweled. The scene was a painting, a postcard, something grand and insig-nificant all at once. From the sky, nothing looked weary or ill. From the sky, there was only potential. I gazed at the highway and tiny toy cars and all the people who didn't know how unlucky they were to be attached to the ground. My face felt bright, lit up like a light bulb. My cheeks hurt from smiling.

Afterward, I continued to show up at the drop zone every weekend. I practiced my skills until I received my solo license, and I made a few hundred more skydives, many of them with Jason. I also figured if I could trust That Guy with my life, we could at least go out on a date. We've been jumping into things together ever since.

THE DECISION TO LIVE WHILE MY MOTHER DIES HAS brought me to the dirty floor of an airport, muddy hiking boots and suitcase wheels near my face. Once Jason leaves, I will be roaming this world alone.

I hug my backpack and wonder if I will be safe, if I will make friends, if I will ever find what my dying mother's restless heart desired. I wonder if this trip will honor my mom or if I am going to rip my family apart. I won-der if I will scurry back to California in just a few weeks or if I will have the resilience to push through when things get tough. My goal is to make it as far as Ha Long Bay, Vietnam—one of the places on my personal bucket list, my measure of success for this journey.

I don't have a lot of money, and my family isn't one of means. I grew up in a small Ohio town, with two significantly older siblings who left home when I was seven. My dad worked his way through the ranks in the air force, and my mom attended job fairs at hotel ballrooms to pick up part-time work whenever things were tight. She took whatever job hired her: she tugged flowers apart at the root and replanted them into plastic flats for nurseries, she ushered people into changing rooms at discount clothing stores, she butchered birds at a turkey farm and came home with spent muscles and rough, cracked fingers.

When I was young, I didn't know we were broke; I thought juice came from cans in the freezer and all toilet paper had only one ply. Later, after my family had moved from working class to solidly middle class, my parents were comfortable enough to help put me through Ohio University with assistance from loans, and the juice in our fridge came from cartons. There wasn't much extra money, though. In college I sold my plasma weekly to afford the luxury of fast food and draft beer, and occasionally I sold chaps and jackets at biker shows for a man named Johnny Marathon, who paid me in cash or leather, my choice. Often I chose wrong.

I worked hard to get things. And now, for this trip, I have sold most everything, including my car and all that old leather. I have a total of $10,000 in the bank and a handshake agreement to write one paid freelance article per month for the newspaper I just left.

Jason is no longer a skydiving instructor; he's a public school teacher, a career change that occurred after we moved to California in 2006. When he returned to college, I said, "At least you'll always have job security. The world always needs teachers," words that have haunted me since the recession in 2008, as Jason has struggled to find a foothold in the system.

A newer teacher, Jason has been laid off every year, then called back as a long-term substitute without benefits and eventually brought back full-time, months into the school year. In 2010, the pink slip came one week before our wedding, when my trip has already been decided. Money is tight enough that we are conscious of every dollar, and there's nothing else to replenish my checking account when the funds are gone.

My international travel experience is limited, and I don't speak any languages beyond English, other than a few sentences from high school French. So if Claude isn't buying socks or headed to the discotheque, I can't help you.

I have no savings, no safety net, and no skills. It's humbling. It's daunting.

I scan the airport and see travelers who look more accomplished, people who wear their courage like a patch across their rugged backpacks. I am not like them. But I close my eyes and remember the words my mother said each day before she sent me off to elementary school: "You are braver than you think."

Back then I was just a girl with long pigtails and a small green backpack, nervous about walking two miles to school on my own. But I wonder if my mom could already look into my brown eyes and see the woman I would become, determined to set off and see the world.

Above us, a speaker crackles and the PA system comes to life. Our plane to Cusco is ready to board.

When You Feel Defeated, Stop to Breathe

———— ⊗⊗⊗ ————

CUSCO FEELS LIKE A PUNCH TO THE CHEST. IT COULD BE that the reality of my jobless, newly homeless, nearly husbandless situation is finally hitting me. Or maybe it's the altitude.

The air in this former Incan capital, perched high in the Andes, is thin and miserly. I have barely stepped off the plane before my asthma causes my lungs to tighten. I anticipated altitude issues until I acclimated to the mountains, but I didn't think they would hit with such force and immediacy. Every inhalation is labored and requires an incredible amount of effort, like trying to blow air into a balloon that has a leak.

After a few puffs on my inhaler, I can breathe easily enough to focus on other things—the wave of tour guides, taxi drivers, hotel operators, and vendors that pushes close as Jason and I make our way through the airport. Sweaty bodies press against us. People tug at our sleeves. Brochures are thrust in our faces. Each person promises a special deal, just for us.

Jason, who has never traveled internationally, looks to me for direction. Of course, I am clueless. Prior to this, I've only traveled outside the United

States on short, easy trips where someone was waiting for me on the other side. But I want to reassure my husband that I am confident and able, a woman who can take care of herself once she is traveling alone.

"Follow me," I say.

Lacking actual experience, I read books instead. I practically memorized the entire "Dangers and Annoyances" section in the Lonely Planet guidebook to Peru. As we navigate the airport, I hiss nuggets of advice to Jason. "Ruthless robberies have been on the rise! Use only official taxis! Hang on to your bag! And remember, do not let anybody share a taxi with us."

Long rows of vendors line the airport hallways. In the middle of one row is a small desk with a wooden sign that says, "Official taxi." The fact that the word "official" is spelled "offecial" barely even registers.

"Are you the official taxi?" I ask.

"*Sí*, we are official taxi," a man behind the desk replies. He motions to the sign and cocks his head, as if to say, *Do you not see this sign? We are clearly offecial.*

"How much?"

"Peruvian?" he says. "Thirty soles."

This is my first time haggling. I don't know how to counter this, other than to say, "Um, no. My guidebook says fifteen soles."

"Ah, but there is an airport tax," he says.

That makes sense. I shrug and hand over the money, the equivalent of twelve dollars.

The man scrawls a handwritten ticket and ushers us outside, directly into another wall of people. He gives our ticket to a different man, who hands it off like a track baton to yet another. It's confusing, and I don't know which man to follow.

"Wait!" I yell.

"This way!" the original vendor points to a car before he is absorbed by the crowd.

I walk to a vehicle that barely qualifies as a car, let alone an official taxi. The driver hoists the backpack off my shoulders and tosses it into the trunk, which is secured shut with a piece of dirty rope. He pushes me toward the open car door, the palm of his hand against my forehead as he shoves me inside. On the other side of the car, the same thing happens to Jason, except with some other Peruvian man we haven't seen before. When Jason sits down, the stranger slides into the seat next to us.

"No," I say. "No strangers in the car."

"Is fine," he says. "I am official taxi."

I whisper "Stranger danger" under my breath, and Jason nods. The driver has already eased the car out of the parking lot and is merging onto a highway. Frequent clicks and pops sound from beneath the taxi. I eye every door—all locked. The back of my neck begins to sweat.

The stranger opens a briefcase on his lap, and I fear we are about to be abducted or given a timeshare pitch. Instead, the stranger hands us photographs. The lamination peels from the corners of each yellowed image.

"How would you like to see Machu Picchu?" he says with all the enthusiasm of a used-car salesman.

I fumble for excuses. "Um, we already have a trek?"

"What about market tour? We take you to alpaca farm, then alpaca shop..."

"No," Jason says.

We have reached the hostel—I recognize the building from the online photos when I booked the place—but the driver continues to circle the block as the salesman piles more photographs into our laps and makes one pitch after another.

"You like party party?" he says.

"No! No party. Please," I beg. "Let us go."

"Ah, you want ancient temple."

Finally, the driver stops the car. In a last-ditch sales effort, the stranger claims he is from the very hostel where we are staying.

"Oh, you're staying at El Tuco?" he says. "I work for El Tuco. Special deal just for you."

Maybe it is the fact that we had been awake for thirty-six hours straight, or maybe the stranger is finally wearing us down. Whatever the cause, Jason and I agree to let him follow us into the hostel while we check in.

I recognize Coco, the owner of El Tuco, also from the photos online. Coco uses his substantial body to fill the front door frame and shouts in Spanish. The stranger mumbles something back. Coco erupts. He screams and takes a step forward, close enough for his breath to make steam on the salesman's face. I anticipate this will come to blows. Instead, the stranger pats his sweaty comb-over and adjusts his shirt, then turns on his heel and marches out the door.

The room is still for a long, awkward beat before I break the silence. "May we check in?" I say. "We're exhausted."

"Check-in is not for three hours," Coco says. "Please sit in the lobby and relax. And welcome to Cusco."

THE NEXT THREE NIGHTS OF OUR HONEYMOON ARE SPENT in a sparsely furnished room at El Tuco that costs eight dollars a night. We sleep on separate foam mattresses, wool hats pulled low over our ears to fight the chill.

"I love you, baby," Jason says from the across the room.

My lips chatter too much to reply.

The windows, lined with iron bars, look out over a highway, a school, and a tightly crammed neighborhood. The room is freezing, but the mold-encrusted shower is excruciatingly hot. I jump in only long enough to boil the germs off my flesh, though I know this will be one of my last hot showers in South America—I should be grateful for water that turns my skin the same color as a ripe tomato.

I have brought an old iPhone on the trip with me, but it's not unlocked and doesn't have a local SIM card, so I can't make regular phone calls. But whenever I'm within range of Wi-Fi, I can hop on the Skype app and make phone calls, either voice or video.

When I call my dad to say I've settled safely in Cusco, I can reach him only on his cell phone. He's at the last place my mom will ever live, a special facility for Alzheimer's patients about thirty miles from the brick house where I grew up. My dad spends hours a day there, every day. Since my mom can no longer walk, he pushes her in a wheelchair around the nursing home, from the parakeet cage in the foyer to the art room where he helps my mom make photo collages and other crafts. He spoons pureed food into her mouth at every meal, because he's convinced the nurses and aides can't do it as well as he can. He knows the other patients who live in the same wing, people who confuse him for a son, a husband, or a brother. He waves and plays along with whatever they say.

When I call, my dad holds the phone up to my mom's ear. I must speak clearly and loudly—her hearing has gone bad—but she doesn't recognize my voice.

"Mom, you would love Cusco. The mountains are so big and green," I say. "Maybe someday I'll bring you here." I know those words are a lie.

The truth is that I'm uneasy talking to her. After a lifetime of conversations, midnight confessions, phone calls from college, I no longer know what to say to my own mom. She offers me little in response, so I don't know if she comprehends anything at all. My words now exist only to fill the blank space. I talk, but for no purpose.

My sister, who lives nearby and visits our mom often, is much better at navigating this territory than I am. She trots out the same conversation you might have with an employee at the post office. "Great weather we're having. I love your sweater. That color makes your eyes pop."

But me, I'm the emotional one, the overthinker. I recall sitting on my mom's lap in her yellow rocking chair, her chin resting on my head as we rocked, a gentle seesaw motion over an ocean of shag carpeting. I was an un-settled child, and my mom soothed me, *shhhh, shhhh*. That is the part I miss most. The comfort. The safe place she built for me. I long for that now: *shhh*. Pulling me close until my heart is against hers.

On the phone my mom mumbles. Her words are gibberish. A sloppy soup of letters. My dad grabs the phone from her.

"Well, kiddo, have a good time. Be safe. You know your mom is very proud of you and loves you."

"Yep. I know." But I don't. My mom hasn't known me in years.

The last time I was in Ohio, several months prior, I sat with my mom in the dining room of her nursing home while she ignored a cup of chocolate pudding. Her once-blonde hair hung limp and gray. Her head lolled against her chest, her eyes downcast. Her face was purple with bruises that she got earlier in the week, a tumble out of her wheelchair when none of the nurses were watching. One doctor suspected my mom had a minor stroke, but it's hard to tell in an unresponsive patient.

A nursing aide tuned a radio to a swing music station and pranced around the room, encouraging the residents to dance. Nobody did. The aide clapped to the music, and it was off beat.

"Mom, I think I'm going to do something really big," I whispered, as I held a spoonful of pudding to her mouth.

She didn't acknowledge my words or my presence.

"Mom, I'm going to travel around the world," I said. When she still didn't move, I put the spoon back into the pudding cup and scooted my chair closer to her wheelchair. I put my hand on her shoulder. Her body went rigid. "If you're in there, you should know I'm doing this for you, okay? If you can't remember anything else, please remember that."

When she finally looked at me, her blue eyes looked past my body, as though I were a potted plant or a utility pole. Her gaze was empty. Then her lips puckered, and she bit at the air, like a baby wanting more. I scooped pudding into her mouth. She glanced up at me, and there was a flash in her watery blue eyes, a moment of awareness that fizzled out as swiftly as it came.

Sometimes I believe my mom is more responsive to me than she is to others, but I don't know if that's a wish, or a lie, or the truth.

When I hang up the phone in Cusco, there's a hollow space carved out of my gut. Unrequited love is always the saddest kind. Sadder still when it's a daughter longing for a mother who no longer recognizes her.

"You okay?" Jason asks.

"I don't know why my dad does that," I say. "She doesn't even know who I am. And she definitely doesn't know I'm gone."

We are interrupted by animal cries punctuating the air outside El Tuco. A market is assembling on the long, slim concrete berm in between lanes of highway traffic, and Jason and I walk outside to investigate. There are cages of squirming puppies and wooden boxes of desiccated fruit, bags of grain, boxes stacked with eggs, blankets piled with wild greens. In the midst of it all, we hear tiny squeals from a mobile guinea pig slaughterhouse.

Guinea pigs—rodents that are neither pig nor from Guinea—are a popular source of protein in Peru, since the animals can be raised quickly in confined spaces. Also, guinea pigs will eat just about anything, which makes them a cheaper form of livestock than cows, pigs, or sheep.

I'm a vegetarian, so I give grilled guinea pig a pass. Instead I've been delighting in Peru's substantial veggie-based options—bowls of buttery quinoa soup, skewers of grilled potato, creamy broad bean stew and slices of crusty brown bread, pale green pepino melons that fit in the palm of my hand.

That night, the dusk that settles over the city is purple. Jason and I sit at a restaurant that looks over the historic buildings of the Plaza de Armas and tuck into *lomo soytado*, a tofu twist on the classic Peruvian *lomo saltado*, in which slivers of beef are stir-fried with peppers, tomatoes, and French fries, all served over rice.

I pretend the rich food and crisp air are making me stronger. But I feel more brittle and unsteady than ever. Each day in Cusco means we are closer to our Inca Trail trek. It's the sensation of standing in the door before my first skydive all over again—slightly sick to my stomach, terrified I won't be able to complete this task, afraid I don't have enough courage. And I'm doing this all for my mom, who doesn't remember I exist.

"Is everything all right?" Jason asks.

Back home in Palm Springs, hiking is one of my favorite activities. I've spent many weekends scrambling over rocks and ambling down dusty desert trails. But that's just something I do for an hour or two before brunch. My hiking doesn't require any real commitment.

In Peru, I realize I've never tackled anything of such a grand scope. They are the high school jocks of mountains—massively and beautifully built, but towering, intimidating, and mean—the stuff of hiking nightmares. Just one look, and you know they are going to hurt you. By comparison, the mountains that encircle my California desert are downright delicate.

"I don't know if I can do this," I admit.

It didn't look so intimidating in the photos or in the piles of travel books on our coffee table. But there in Cusco, just looking at the peaks and spires of granite makes me want to cry. I can't imagine four straight days of navigating their peaks with my own two feet. I feel like I've just shown up at the start line for a marathon after only watching the Olympics on TV. What was I thinking?

Beyond that, I am ill. I feel like I should have acclimated already, but after three days in Cusco I am still beset with altitude sickness. Even walking short distances causes me to clutch my chest, fumbling for my inhaler on Cusco's fierce, sloped streets. When I'm not wheezing, I am trying to locate the nearest toilet for my upset stomach.

"Of course you can do this," Jason says, and he hands over my extra inhaler, which he has tucked away in his pocket. "You've jumped out of airplanes, right? You can handle a little walk."

The Inca Trail is hardly a little walk, but I don't want to dwell on that. Jason has been looking forward to the trek more than any other part of our honeymoon. I can't disappoint him, especially when I'm about to leave him for a year.

"Of course I can handle a little walk," I say.

THE EVENING BEFORE THE HIKE, JASON AND I MAKE FINAL preparations. We separate our belongings into what is necessary and what we can leave behind.

My backpack is a hefty, fifty-pound clown car of everything I anticipate needing for my entire trip—paperback novels, a laptop, sleeping bag, first aid kit, electrical outlet adapter, vitamins, a flashlight, whistle, water sterilizer, tofu jerky, shampoo, duct tape, T-shirts, tights, dresses, jeans, two fleece jackets, one iPhone, a slim towel, and four pairs of shoes. For four days on the Inca Trail, however, only a few things qualify as necessities. Everything else can be stored in a locker at El Tuco while we are away.

Our necessities include a toothbrush, designer wool socks, several layers of fancy, sweat-wicking clothing, and ridiculous hiking poles that cost almost as much as a car payment. This was magical thinking on my part; I imagined the more expensive the equipment, the easier it would make the trek.

We have already gone through most of our clean socks and underwear. El Tuco doesn't have any laundry facilities, and we haven't found a Laundromat nearby, so I use a hard-bristled brush and hand soap to scrub our dirty clothes in the bathroom sink. Jason stretches a portable clothesline from one corner of the room to the other. There aren't any nails or hooks in the wall, so he cracks the window enough to tie the line around the iron bars. When he does this, I shiver. It's July, the start of winter in South America. The mountain air has sharp teeth, especially at night.

Jason and I pack and repack, adding and subtracting items, searching for the perfect equation—all the things we want to carry on our backs for twenty-six miles, still keeping it light enough that we won't be tempted to toss anything off the side of a mountain. I am delirious with sleep deprivation and altitude sickness; I decide to bring eyeliner but leave behind toothpaste.

I rub my eyes. It's already midnight, and our bus is scheduled to pick us up at 5 a.m. I flop on the hard bed and cover myself with a thin blanket.

"I'm done. I can't pack any more. Whatever we have now, that's what we're bringing," I say. "I need sleep."

"Yeah, I'm wiped out," Jason agrees. "And we have mountains to climb."

He reaches for the socks and underwear, still hanging on the clothesline, the final addition to our packs before we can go to bed.

"Uh oh," he says.

"What? Don't uh oh."

I stand and touch the clothes on the sagging line. The socks are wet and cold, the underwear frozen stiff. There's no way these things will dry in time for our hike.

Frustration coils through my limbs, and I kick my bag, spilling all the things I had so carefully packed.

"Maybe they'll dry by the time the bus gets here …?"

The laundry has been hanging for hours. If it isn't dry by now, it will never be dry. That's it. Our hike is ruined before it even began. The failure feels inevitable.

Jason runs downstairs to ask the front desk if there is a twenty-four-hour Laundromat anywhere in the vicinity. He returns several minutes later with one of his hands hidden behind his back. With a magician's flourish, he holds his right hand out and presents to me a miniature travel hair dryer.

"I borrowed it from an Irish couple down the hall," he says. "They said we can just leave it outside their door when we're done."

Two hours later, the underwear is dry, but I am still blowing a weak shaft of hot air into the woolen toes of thick socks. Each time the hair dryer overheats, we have to wait a few minutes for it to start again. I teeter on the edge of hysteria, and I lash out at my husband.

"Why did I buy such nice socks? This never would have happened with my normal, shitty socks. Some of my old socks even have holes. I bet those would've dried real quick. But these things?" I say, getting louder and more forceful with every sentence. "Fuck these socks! Fuck it all. Fuck the Inca Trail . . ."

"Shhh," Jason eases an arm around me and pries the hair dryer away with the other. "Let me dry these for a while. You rest."

The action is small but tender and represents everything I love about this man. Where I gripe and complain, Jason is thoughtful, nurturing, supportive. For years I thought marriage was incompatible with the life I wanted to lead as an independent woman, but here is my husband, comforting me in an eight-dollar-a-night hostel, proving otherwise. What the hell am I doing leaving him on purpose? Leaving my career and my home and my dying mother? And for what? Wet socks and granite mountains?

I'm filled with a sudden longing for my mom. She was always protective. I remember how my elementary school gym teacher never let me visit the school nurse for a puff of my inhaler before gym class. Then came the day I collapsed on a dry, weed-strewn field. I awoke on a couch in the nurse's office, my mom holding my hand and smoothing the hair from my forehead. She slid one hand behind my head and helped me tilt forward to take a puff from the emergency inhaler she kept tucked in her purse. Then my mom whispered stories until my pulse slowed and the weight on my lungs disappeared. When it was clear that I'd recovered, my mom tracked down the gym teacher and unleashed her rage on the man, hissing, "How dare you make little girls suffer? What kind of man are you?"

I can't recall exactly how the situation was resolved—whether I was pulled from that teacher's class or if he was ever punished. The implication, though, has remained my entire life. My husband has done his share of time comforting me, but it is my mom who always soothed me when I gasped for air.

As a child I was a sickly thing, hospitalized more than once for asthma attacks and vicious bouts of pneumonia and bronchitis. My mom stayed by my side, even when nurses tried to shoo her away. She was there to hold my hand, her strong fingers wrapped around my tiny ones, through the night and until things were right again. I wish she could do that now.

Nobody warned me about this part. When I envisioned my trip, I imagined exciting adventures, exotic locales, a jet-set lifestyle. I never thought grief and doubt would climb into my backpack and come with me. I pictured standing at the top of the Sun Gate, looking down at Machu Picchu, without ever thinking about the steps it would take to get there. This is the curse of wanderlust, when the postcard image becomes a brutal reality.

All the exhaustion, sickness, and worry that has been tipping me for days finally knocks me over. I collapse in quiet sobs on the bed, swallowing deep gulps of air. Jason holds me until I calm, then fall asleep.

The wake-up alarm sounds after just two hours, and Jason and I rub our bleary eyes as we step onto a bus.

Soon the sun will rise over the Andes, and we will be there to welcome it. Our socks are dry. A mountain invites us to climb it.

Push Yourself Until
You Can't Turn Back

―――⚬⚬⚬―――

OUR FIRST HIKING DAY ON THE INCA TRAIL TREK IS SUP-
posed to be the easiest. But our guide, Juan, jokingly calls it "Inca flat,"
meaning it is not flat at all.

For several miles we walk undulating roller-coaster hills that never seem
to wane. We keep pace with the rest of our group, though, which consists of
two other honeymooning couples, an older outdoorsman from Oregon, and
a grandmotherly type.

Along the way we see hikers from other groups splinter off, turning
around to head back to the station at the base of the mountain in Sacred
Valley. Some are visibly sick, their heads lolling and sleepy-eyed, their bodies
draped over donkeys as they are led to the start of the trail. Some have just
realized for the first time how brutal the hike can be.

"That's the problem," Juan says. "You never know if you can handle the
trail until you try."

I realize then there's no easy way out. There is no evacuation plan.

If the trail breaks me, my choices are limited to going back where I came from or pushing forward to the end. Each mile all of a sudden feels incredibly real.

Groups of traditionally dressed Peruvian women sit by the side of the trail, selling cans of beer and bottles of energy drinks. In a moment of weakness my husband pays Disneyland prices for a small bottle of Gatorade. It is delicious.

My group makes it to the first night's campsite intact, though my arms are salty and a layer of skin on my heel has already sloughed off in my hiking shoes.

The porters, who all jogged ahead of us, are waiting. While we were huffing our way to camp, they erected the tents and prepared a feast of brown bread, quinoa stew, fresh salad, and grilled alpaca steaks. It is a guilty relief.

We eat in a large dining tent, lit by small lanterns. After a day of sweat and effort, my body is sore and cold. I warm my hands around a metal cup of hot chocolate.

When we've finished dinner, Juan ushers us to our nearby campsite.

"You've been to a four-star hotel, eh?" he asks. "Well, welcome to your thousand-star hotel."

Our campsite is just past the small town of Wayllabamba, tucked away on a grassy, terraced hillside deep in the Andes Mountains. With stone structures and layers of mountain, it looks like a mini Machu Picchu. We've hiked beyond many of the other groups on the trail and are camping in a secluded spot at a higher elevation, but I see the rounded mushroom tops of other tents below, shocking bursts of primary colors in between the green of the landscape.

As the night settles, the sky is heaped with stars dripping down in strands that nearly touch the tops of our tents. It is more magnificent than a Ritz, more dazzling than a fancy Hilton. The tent door is unzipped, and the inside looks inviting. The sleeping bags are fat and red, almost plushy. My muscles relax just at the sight of this.

When I pause outside my tent and take a deep breath, I am surprised to get a lung full of air, bracing and crisp as green apples. We are still miles from where we need to go. But for now, I can breathe.

AT 5 A.M., MY TENT IS UNZIPPED AND THE SMALL FACE OF the assistant guide, Pedro, peeks through the flap.

"*Café* or *té?*"

"Both. Either. Anything."

When Pedro pushes a hot tin cup my way, I am groggy enough that I don't pay any mind to what I'm drinking until I'm almost finished. That's when I realize I've had my first coca tea, made using the raw leaves of the coca plant. Though the plant is the source of cocaine, the coca leaves themselves are only a mild stimulant and are often used to soothe altitude sickness. The taste is grassy and herbal but slightly sweeter than green tea.

"Jason, I feel like my cells are dancing," I say.

My eyes widen and there's a new zing in my movements. I dress in about three seconds and am ready for what promises to be the roughest day of hiking, the day we will tackle Dead Woman's Pass.

The undulating hills are long gone. This morning's hike is all about gaining altitude. The path is steep, set with wide, heavy slabs of stone, and there are no plateaus to offer relief. Every step takes excruciating effort, and I often have to squat to catch my breath.

At almost 14,000 feet and sucking in at least 30 percent less oxygen at this altitude, it feels like I'm inflating balloons while climbing a never-ending staircase. Before long, I am passed by every member of my group, then hikers from other groups. Even llamas go by.

"This is dumb," I say to my husband. "There are buses that go up to Machu Picchu."

"But there are things we can only see from the trail," Jason says. "And we wanted to see Machu Picchu the same way the Incas did, remember?"

"I am not an Inca," I mutter.

Jason is right, though. The trail has magnificent views, especially today's section, as we climb from the valley floor through the moist forest and into the greenest mountains I have ever seen.

This is a highway, constructed more than 500 years ago. Like all old highways, it's deeply cracked, with branching fissures that look like a circulatory system in the stone. Orchids, grasses, and plants erupt through the rifts. Their roots go deep; their blooms shoot high. Wisps of cloud float overhead, just passing by.

All day long I have my eye on Dead Woman's Pass—so called because the mountain ridge resembles the silhouette of a supine woman—but the pass never seems to get any closer. Jason takes my backpack and murmurs words of encouragement.

"You're a superstar. You're the best hiker in the world," he says, but I can barely hear him. My pulse throbs in my ears, and I pant like a hound dog.

"I don't know if I'll make it," I say.

I remember the night we decided to make Peru our honeymoon destination. I brought home *Where to Go When*, a coffee table book filled with glossy, vibrant photos of far-flung places. The book is divided into months, listing the best places to visit and the best things to do during that period of time. Jason and I knew we wanted to honeymoon in summer, so we separately flipped through the June, July, and August sections and made a list of our top five places. When we traded our lists, both of us had the same thing written in the number-one slot: Machu Picchu.

I remembered my mom putting the ruins high on her bucket list too. She never quite said the name correctly. "Mushu Picchu. Mashu Pizza. You know what I mean," she'd say with a cascading laugh.

After planning, dreaming, and saving, Jason and I are finally on our way. I am ascending a mountain with the man I love, and I can see the peak from where I stand. I'm crazy to even think about turning back.

The final push to Dead Woman's Pass is a 3,000-foot elevation gain over the course of three hours. It feels like an exercise machine set for the highest level, like one of those stair-climbers that never take you anywhere. My joints ache from the force of being yanked uphill and into motion while the altitude tries to smash me down. I look to my feet for several minutes, then I focus on the hairy calves of the man in front of me, then I stare at the sky, then back to the ground. My lungs feel like fire.

After about an hour, I enter a Zen-like meditation, in which I count my steps and allow the numbers to fill my head. "One, two, three … ugh, four, five, six …" Every time I get to 250, I start over. I don't know why I decided to focus on numbers, but it helps. It gives me a focus beyond the struggle to breathe and walk; it takes me beyond the trail. It's kind of like having an out-of-body experience, though if I were out of my body then my thighs wouldn't burn so much.

Eventually, there is a moment when my feet are moving but I no longer have to force myself to climb. I am simply doing it.

When I reach the top of the pass, I stop staring at my shoes, at the ground, at the unyielding sky. From this vantage point, the highest point of this hike, I see snow-capped peaks. Miles of mountains, embroidered with gray trails. And my hiking group, waiting for me. All I hear is applause.

I've made it.

By the end of the day, after a brief descent to our campsite, we are closer to the end of the trail than the beginning. We've gone too far to turn back.

DAY THREE PROMISES TO BE LONG—NEARLY TEN MILES total—but we are given motivation for hiking faster and harder than ever. Showers wait for us at the campsite, the first opportunity to bathe on this trek.

Juan also says the first group to the campsite will have a better position on the trail the following morning, the day we will finally see Machu Picchu.

Along the way, we walk the same path the Inca paved, with many of the original stones still in place. We pause for breakfast at Runkuracay, small, circular ruins made of stone, which overlook the Pacamayo valley. We hike along steep rock embankments, skirting deep precipices.

Another set of ruins is called Sayacmarca, "inaccessible town," protected by sheer cliffs on three sides. The structures remain secretive—nobody knows exactly why they were built and how they were used—and I am overwhelmed. There are stories here, fossilized in the buildings, and nobody can ever unearth them. How can something be both tangible and so unknown?

This is my mom's narrative. She still exists, but her stories are lost forever. Her death is the kind that she is forced to live every day, paused somewhere between earth and what exists beyond. She is my inaccessible town.

I scramble to hold fast to my memories of my mom, but time has faded them. I remember bits and snapshots: Our overgrown backyard in Huber Heights, Ohio, where my mom let me run through the garden sprinkler, though she somehow never got wet. Afternoon walks to the duck pond, tossing stale crusts to the birds. Picking wild mulberries in the woods, staining our hands the color of a bruise. Pushing me on a swing my brother hung from the maple tree in the front yard; I know one day the swing fell, but I can't remember if she caught me.

One time my plastic digital watch stopped working, and my mom slapped it across her palm with such force it turned her hand pink. "Just needs a good German touch," she said as the digital numbers reappeared.

I have wispy memories of her when she was slender and tall, swishing into the house after attending grown-up parties. I purposely stayed awake long after the babysitter put me to bed, just to receive my mom's soft kiss on my forehead. I relished the vision of her draped in sparkly jewelry, dressed elegantly, illuminated by a shaft of moonlight, the sweet smell of a strawberry daiquiri mixed with perfume. Why should that vibrant version of my mom exist only in the past?

If I shut my eyes, I can resurrect her; when I open them again, she is lost.

When I sniffle, Jason stops. "What's wrong?" he says, and he pushes a lock of sweaty hair from my forehead.

We're so close to the finish line of this spectacular place, the end of the goal we set for our honeymoon hike. Soon he'll return to California, and I'll continue wandering, with no clear-cut path. It's hard enough for me to keep going when there's a trail pointing the way. How am I supposed to keep going when there is nobody to guide me? Will I be strong enough to carry myself?

"Nothing's wrong," I say. "I just don't want this trail to come to an end."

We're at a place where the path is broken and uneven, where many of the original stones are coming undone. The rocks are hard but unstable. Stairs crumble beneath our feet. The air is moist, and most steps are covered with slippery, wet leaves, so every movement requires extra vigilance. This feels like the most treacherous ground of all. I feel most unsteady.

After a few more hours of hiking through the cloud forest, we finally reach our campsite for the night, Wiñay Wayna, named for the pink orchid that grows only here. In Quechua, the indigenous language, it means "forever young."

Our tents are erected near an extensive set of Incan ruins—agricultural terraces, house-like structures, walkways with long staircases and large baths.

This is where I take my first shower in three days. I pay $1.50 for three minutes of hot water. I feel as though I've been baptized, reborn through this age-old ritual of walking, sweating, scrubbing the dirt from my feet, becoming clean again.

PEDRO WAKES THE GROUP AT 4 A.M.

"Let's go, let's go. *Arriba!*"

We are given coffee and thin, rolled crepes for breakfast, which we eat in silence. This is going to be the easiest day of hiking, only about three hours until we reach the Sun Gate, but the sense of ending is palpable. Today we will see Machu Picchu, and then we will scatter on our own ways.

It is dark outside, the kind of dark when dawn seems unreachable. With flashlights in hand, we take to the trail. The goal is to get to the ruins before sunrise, but Juan warns that we must be careful. At this point the path is a delicate contour that winds a thin line around the mountains, with sheer drop-offs to the right. Juan says some hikers have tumbled from the trail and were only discovered weeks later.

We walk single file, with Juan following close behind.

"Mountainside!" he hisses when any of us stray too far to the edge.

When I look backward, I see scores of other hikers and their flashlights, like a string of Christmas lights draped along the Andes.

Before long we hit an official checkpoint, where a guard must check our

Inca Trail hiking permits (the trail is limited to 500 hikers and porters per day, and this is strictly regulated) and stamp our passports. However, the office doesn't open until 5:30 a.m.—we still have more than an hour to wait. Juan didn't tell us about this part.

It is cold, and Jason and I huddle together for warmth.

"Aw, it's like being on the floor of the Lima airport all over again, honey," I say.

"Stop."

We try to pass the time with games, but even the woman who was once a cruise ship entertainer—a bubbly, chatty blonde—has lost her natural enthusiasm.

"I spy something with my little eye," she mutters. Her scarf is bundled around her face. She sits on a bench near the guard's office and looks more like a heap of blankets than a person.

"Is it black?" I say.

"Yes."

"Is it darkness?"

"Yes. You win. Game over."

The guard arrives and checks our documents. As soon as he gives us the proper stamps, we sprint. The last hour is all running. I take puffs from my emergency inhaler as we jog higher and higher.

Finally, as dawn breaks, we reach the final ascent. Fifty steps, nearly vertical. The angle is so dramatic, I'm forced to approach it like a child and climb on my hands and feet in a bear crawl.

When I reach the top, I look down and gasp. It's there. Machu Picchu, all spread out below me. It's like a massive Lego masterpiece—a dazzling display of carefully laid blocks, precise stone architecture, and staircases of terraces hewn from the rich green land.

There are places that never live up to the hype. There are places that will never look as good as the postcards. Machu Picchu is not one of those places. It's there, I see it, but it doesn't look possible.

This is where the Andes Mountains meet the Amazon Basin in a tropical mountain forest. The velvety mountaintops look like rococo sculptures, draped with valances of mosses, dotted with ferns, decorated by canopies of trees. It is an embarrassment of green. Wispy fog forms gauzy rings around each peak.

About 200 structures form the sanctuary of Machu Picchu, set on steep ridges of granite and laced with white rock terraces. The walls of each building are formed so perfectly that a knife cannot be wedged in between the stones. Llamas graze nearby. Jason and I sit and watch the sun move across the mountains, our eyes clouded with tears. A flock of neon green parakeets swoops overhead.

I think of my mom now, as I take in this place I didn't know I was strong enough to reach. She would be proud of the four days I spent breathing in sun, the nights spent sleeping among stars. She'd want to see me here, strong in the midst of ruins.

I wonder if the wounds we carry inside us are like the wounds we show on the outside. I remember falling often as a clumsy little girl, all scabbed knees and elbows. My mother was slow to bandage me. Instead she told me to give my cuts sunshine and air, the necessary ingredients to heal.

Maybe this is what brought me to Peru at this particular moment. She has been sick for ten years. I know my mom's death is coming, and that wound is raw and vulnerable. But Machu Picchu is a reminder of timelessness. Even when abandoned, it wasn't destroyed. Some things never disappear.

The sun is round and bright as Jason and I scramble among the buildings, feeling the polished stones laid by fifteenth-century hands. A breeze spills over the mountains and rolls down the terraces. We clamber up a hill to a carved pillar called Intihuatana, which translates to "the hitching post of the sun." It's a sundial of sorts, where Incan astronomers once predicted the celestial periods. On the vernal and autumnal equinoxes each year, the sun halts over the pillar at midday, casting no shadow.

Those are the days when the sun has lassoed the rock, and for the briefest, most golden moment, the earth and sky meet. Once separated, the two spend the next six months traveling the universe to find each other again.

I kneel by the pillar and put my hand atop the rock. It is still warm.

You're Not Lost. The Trail Is.

JASON AND I ARRIVE ON A SMALL AIRCRAFT FOR THE SEC-ond part of our honeymoon and are whisked immediately onto a small metal boat. We are several miles from Iquitos, the world's largest city that cannot be accessed by roads. Jesus, our guide to the rainforest, deftly ties the boat to an old stump near the edge of the Amazon River.

Looking around the jungle that now surrounds us, Jason whispers, "What is this world?" He's staring at a tree that appears to be filled with flowers until the blooms move and shake. Parakeets. They seem to take flight simultaneously, one enormous, fluttery cloud blotting out the sky above.

"It's magic," I whisper back.

We walk up a small slope into a thick ribbon of trees. I'm just about ten steps under the rainforest canopy when Jesus hisses, "Stop and back away slowly."

My right foot, which had been poised to step, now hangs midair. This is our first afternoon in the Amazon, but I already know enough to treat the word of Jesus like the word of, well, Jesus. I awkwardly shuffle to my left foot. My hiking boots make a soggy, suction-cup sound as I retreat in the mud.

"You see that snake?" Jesus says.

"No."

"Look carefully." He points. "Very dangerous."

I scrutinize the area that surrounds my boot prints. Under the thick canopy of trees, the forest is almost completely dark. I see mud, and I see rotting brown leaves. What I don't see is a snake.

"You still don't see? The snake that was going to bite you?" When I shake my head no, Jesus sighs.

He waits for the snake to move, and that's when I finally see the reptile's firm, oval head. It startles me, even though I already know he's there. He slithers away, disappearing beneath fleshy green plants.

We continue into the forest. This time, though, I eye the trail nervously. There are things here that could kill me. Things that probably want to kill me. I feel vulnerable in a way I've never felt back in California, among the gated housing developments and landscaped golf courses. I'd seen wildlife at home, sure. Coyotes, lizards, and snakes. They were there first, and they made regular appearances as a reminder. But at least I felt empowered on familiar terrain.

I don't have high hopes for my survival in this topsy-turvy place, where trees blot out the sky and the roads are made of rivers. I don't know how to find my way out of the forest, back to the boat, and down the river to the lodge where Jason and I are staying. If I'm being honest, I don't even know how to pronounce the name of the lodge where we are staying.

I love this new, unfamiliar territory, though.

I remember joining a save-the-rainforest initiative when I was in the sixth grade. I threw myself wholeheartedly into the effort. I stopped eating meat because I read cattle farms were a major cause of deforestation. I signed petitions. I wrote letters to President Reagan. I rattled off facts about conserving the rainforest, wrote reports about it for school. I wore "Save the Rainforest" T-shirts emblazoned with tree frogs. My mom was proud of my passion.

Yet, while I knew about the dangers facing the rainforest, I didn't know much about the rainforest itself. I hadn't expected the funhouse mirror where I am standing now, a place where everything is distorted, lovely and strange. Pink river dolphins leap through the water. Snakes grow as thick as tree trunks, and lily pads are as large and round as Volkswagen Beetles. Lizards and frogs flicker with neon color. Tiny, shrunken monkeys slingshot through the treetops. The moist air feels like light rain.

It is a magnificent but intimidating landscape. Each day my heart pounds as the three of us—Jesus, Jason, and I—venture deeper into the forest. It is warm, dark, and slippery, like descending into a massive throat.

"Hey, Jesus, did I tell you about the rainforest club I was in when I was a little girl?" I say. "We wrote petitions and recycled cans and raised money to save the rainforest."

"Looks like it worked," he says. "Good job."

This is his land, where Jesus was born and raised. His body is lean, brown, and agile. His eyes are rainforest trained. He knows every tree like it's his neighbor. He can see poisonous snakes when I can't. He even finds a path where there is seemingly none.

I examine the ground beneath my feet. There isn't a path below us.

"Uh, Jesus, did you notice there's no trail anymore?"

"Mmm-hmm."

I tug on Jesus's shirtsleeve, pulling him to a stop, and I look around.

"Seriously. Are we lost?"

Jesus turns and stares at me without blinking.

"No, we're not lost. We're right here," he says. "The trail is lost."

Then he continues walking, leaving his own tracks in the inch-deep mud. I follow him and have faith the trail will come to us.

After an hour, we come to a clearing where a series of stout wooden poles, ropes, and ladders lead into the air. Jesus urges me to climb one of the ladders. Jason follows.

The ladder leads to a rope bridge, strung high above the treetops. We emerge from the crinoline band of mist into limitless clear blue air. From this vantage, I look down on blooming orchids curling through tree branches, scarlet macaws in flight against towers of clouds. From here I can see no path at all. Just the wide, open world, waiting for me to explore it. I think about that old quote, "Not all who wander are lost," and it feels true.

I'm not lost. I'm right here. The path might become obscured or disappear entirely, but I'm still where I belong.

That night Jason and I sleep in a thatched hut. Fear wakes me in the deepest, most aggressive point of night. At first I'm unclear on what has gripped me, why I am no longer asleep, what is holding my throat closed. Then I realize the gauzy mosquito net above the bed has fallen across my head and into my mouth. I claw at my face, push the netting away.

Too shaken to rest, I curl into a corner and turn on my headlamp. There is a cloud of bugs illuminated by the beam of light. I wave them away the best I can, then focus on reading a couple of chapters in a book, enough to make me tired again.

After I crawl under the sheets, I tuck the edge of the mosquito net under the mattress and settle back against Jason. His body rises and falls with every breath, asleep. He didn't even notice I was gone, and this comforts me. Maybe it's possible to stray from his side and return home again, no damage done. I don't know how true this is, though.

Holding a family together is hard. The first time I understand this is also the first time I am distinctly aware that something is wrong with Mom. I am twenty-one or maybe twenty-two. I believe myself to be a grown-up, even though I'm at home for the weekend to have my dad change the oil in my car. My mom hasn't been diagnosed yet, but that doesn't mean everything is okay.

She is crying. It is such a rare thing to see my mom cry that I don't know what to do. It's like watching a puppy cry. I want to make everything better, but I am powerless. My dad is frustrated, pleading with her to listen.

She has papers. Lists. Scribbled notes about every person who called our landline over the past few months. Men and women. She believes the women are calling my dad for sex, the men are part of the hookup. It's a sex ring, maybe. It's an orgy, probably.

My dad has never been unfaithful. I know this.

Exasperated, my dad pulls me into their argument. I've never been privy to the inner workings of their marriage before, and now I am submerged. We sit at the kitchen table, me acting as the mediator, and suddenly I don't feel grown-up at all. My mom says she and my dad haven't been making love; it has been a long time since she was desired. She is growing old and feels unloved and believes she is going to die alone, and meanwhile these people keep calling. *Why are they calling?!* The people on the other end say they are wrong numbers, but she is confident they are lying.

They are wrong numbers. This is something else I know.

The local Big Lots once published our phone number instead of their own. The mistake was corrected as soon as it was discovered, but the damage was already done. Our line has received years of wrong numbers. They came frequently enough that I learned the Big Lots store hours; it is easier to give people what they want than explain why they are wrong.

Comforting my mom, I learn that lesson all over again. I can't say her piles of notes frighten me and that I think she's going crazy, but I can't indulge her stories either. So I don't tell her she's wrong; I also don't tell her she's right. I only reassure her.

Of course the phone calls are unsettling, I say. Of course dad still loves you. He always has. Of course you're not old. Of course you are still lovable. Of course you are not going to die alone. You are not going to die.

It is a precarious thing to hold a family together, an elaborate system of knots and lines.

Eventually the argument changes from a rapid boil to a low simmer. My dad goes to bed. My mom sits in the yellow rocking chair in the living room, rocking back and forth in the darkness. There is one electric candle in the window, and the glow from that casts an eerie shadow over her face. I go to her. I'm too big to sit on her lap, but I try to hold her anyway. She scoots the chair so that I cannot.

"Just go," she says. "Leave me alone."

This is one of the last things I remember her saying to me.

Right now in the Amazon, my limbs are warm where the insects have chewed my skin, and I already feel lumps forming in response. The itch is maddening. But this also provides its own strange comfort. If my heart is going to hurt all the way around the world, my flesh might as well feel it too.

Earlier today, Jason and I paused on that suspension bridge across the rainforest canopy. I was somewhere near the middle, but Jason hung back at the beginning. He might be a skydiver, but he is also afraid of heights like this—edges and ledges and bridges, the kind of heights where you are certain how high you are.

He took one tentative step toward me. His hands gripped the ropes on either side until his knuckles bulged.

"Don't look down," I said.

He took a few more steps. Baby ones. As his confidence built, his hands loosened. For one moment, he didn't hold on to anything. He moved forward with the trust that the bridge would hold.

That's when I jumped up and down. I shook the whole thing for no good reason.

Sleep Always Comes

⚬⚬⚬

SEVERAL DAYS LATER, JASON AND I ARE BACK IN LIMA. IT is Fiestas Patrias, when Peruvians celebrate their independence. Revelers dance and shout on the street, and the discos stay open well past dawn. Jason and I walk around the city as long as we can bear to be around other people; then we retreat to our hotel. It is our last night together.

Our hotel is a place that looks like a dollhouse, a tiny wooden structure painted in vivid green, red, and yellow. It's perched on the roof of an apartment building in Barranco, an artsy section of downtown Lima. The rooftop is crowded with wooden awnings and climbing vines, potted palms, a cage full of finches, wind chimes made of seashells. Jason and I warm our hands at the fire pit and drink dark Peruvian beer from the bottle. From the rooftop, it's easy to feel removed from the rest of this world, as if the thing I've been dreading will never happen.

"I don't want you to go," I say.

"I don't want to go either, but we knew this was part of it," Jason says. "I have to go away in order to get you back home again."

I have a hat woven from alpaca wool, a gift Jason bought from one of the vendors at the Independence Day festival. I pull it down over my icy ears. I am cold, cold all over, like my blood has stopped moving.

We could go out and dance our fears away. We could get completely smashed and forget that we won't be able to hold each other again for one year. Instead, we step inside our dollhouse, this perfectly constructed toy version of a home, and burrow into bed. We cling to each other, making love on itchy blankets. When I cry, my tears roll down his bare shoulders.

Jason decides we should pretend he's not leaving in the morning, so we try to create some sense of normalcy. There's a small TV near the bed, and we wiggle the knobs until we find something that reminds us of home: *Los Simpsons*. We split another beer and laugh at the show, even though we have no idea what the characters are saying.

We are smiling, but the moment feels false. I know what's coming. I can't tune out the fact that I'm going to spend tomorrow—and 364 more tomorrows—without him.

Jason holds me close to his body until I fall asleep, but I never make it to a dream state, and the rest of the night feels half-lived. My eyes are closed, but I hear the throbbing bass of the music at the discotheque. I wish I could run downstairs and lose myself in the noisy ocean of people, so I wouldn't have to live through the loss I've constructed for myself.

In the morning, the cab arrives right on schedule. Jason gives me a kiss and walks out the door, as if he's leaving for work. I punch the pillow and shove my face in the divot. Keki, the Peruvian woman who owns the bed-and-breakfast, creeps up the stairs and leaves a tray of food. I don't want it. I don't want anything but a flight back to California with Jason, and a mom who isn't dying, and a family that feels whole again.

Keki grows concerned when I don't leave the dollhouse for a full day. The following morning she tries to bring me breakfast. Today it's coffee and a dry pastry. I can't imagine trying to choke it down my sad, raw throat.

"He's gone," she says. "Now you must continue. The year will pass quickly. Come on, you are stronger than this."

Her words sound like a mother's scolding, and they remind me of how

I've already accomplished things on this trip I never thought I could do. I made it to Dead Woman's Pass. I've crept past snakes in the Amazon. Surely I can get dressed and go outside. Keki gives me directions to a vegetarian restaurant inside an old train car, a place known to be lively with young people.

"Will make you happy," she says.

The restaurant doesn't make me happy. There are couples at every table, piles of couples upon couples, and I feel woefully alone. I know the idea of this trip was to assert my independence, to blaze my own path while honoring the one my mother couldn't take for herself, but now it feels stupid and simple. Worse, I wonder if I'm even allowed to feel this sad over a decision I made.

When the waiter comes to my table, I order quinoa soup, and then I begin to cry. I remember the quinoa soup Jason and I ate on the Inca Trail, the way the rich broth warmed me, the way we delighted over the simple flavors.

The waiter leans over me and looks puzzled, which only makes me cry harder.

"My husband left me," I say. I consider trying to explain further. I could tell him that this was all part of a plan. That I am not getting a divorce. That this is me, asserting my place in the world while coming to terms with the profound loss of my mother. But those words won't make any sense, and they don't matter anyway. The truth of this moment is that my husband left me. I am alone. That is what's real.

"What can I do?" the helpless waiter asks. Nothing. He can't do anything for me.

I return to the dollhouse, thank Keki for her kindness and generosity, and carefully pack my backpack. Peru is like an amber stone, suspending all the beautiful memories of my honeymoon with Jason. I can't look at it any longer. It's time to head to Bolivia.

I BOARD A BUS IN THE MORNING, UNSURE OF WHAT AWAITS me. Before I cross into Bolivia, I pause in the border town of Puno. The region is all dry plains and pale grasses that stop short at the shore of Lake Titicaca.

The lake is magnificent, expansive and dramatic, like looking out over a still ocean. The water is the color of the sky at home in Palm Springs, a fierce, ferocious blue. Unapologetic. At once I am entranced at the purity of this place; I have never seen anything so clear before. I want to grab fistfuls of water, carry it around in my pocket, save it.

Of course, I can't. But I can stay here for a few days and soak it in with my eyes.

At a nearby hostel, I ask about the islands of the lake. The most popular destination for tourists is Los Uros, floating islands constructed from totora reeds. The residents here are the Uros, the pre-Incan people—some legends even claim they are older than the sun.

Nobody knows exactly when the Uros moved into the middle of the lake, just that they have lived there for centuries on land they created with the cattail-type reeds, which rot and must be replaced regularly with more reeds. Now only a few hundred Uros remain full-time on the islands, where they live in thatched houses, also made from totora. The majority of the Uros have moved to the mainland.

I'm interested in the more populated islands in Lake Titicaca, each of which functions like an autonomous country with its own rules, governing body, and culture.

Isla Taquile, once seized by the Incan empire in the fifteenth century, is now a small island populated with about 2,000 Taquileños who speak Quechua and Spanish. Most of the men speak Quechua, and most of the women speak Spanish, which is baffling but fascinating. I've always marveled at how relationships work, especially when the individuals seem to combine like oil and water. My mom and my dad, for instance, are such different people—he's hard-nosed and loud; she's soft and quick with a golden laugh. If you saw them in a room full of people, you'd never make that match.

My father grew up among the alfalfa and cornfields of small-town Indiana, a jock who entered the U.S. Air Force just out of high school. He learned about the world through military deployments. On the other hand, my mother's birthplace is no longer a country. Her family left East Prussia during World War II, then worked their way toward what was then known as West Germany, where they finally settled. As a child, she picked potatoes to feed her family.

My dad met my mom in Germany, where she was working as a civilian secretary at Sembach Air Force Base, where he was stationed. With their marriage, two cultures intertwined.

Isla Taquile is full of those confounding relationships—couples who make it work even when they don't inhabit the same language.

The hilly island, roped with gray paths, is distinctive for a few other reasons: It has no police, no prison, and no dogs (which are viewed as a sign of security). The island does not have cars or electricity. Running water is rare. The people follow just three laws: *Ama sua. Ama llulla. Ama qhilla.* Do not steal. Do not lie. Do not be lazy.

Even more appealing to me is that the people of Taquile eat a plant-based diet. I've had some terrific meals in Peru, but so many of the vegetarian dishes are exactly the same: French fries, omelets, quinoa soup, brown bread. Though the Taquile people supplement their diet with trout from the lake, they are mostly vegetarian. I expect their food to be inventive and delicious, using the agricultural gifts of the island—something beyond eggs, fried potatoes, and bread.

My intention is to do a homestay for at least one night on the island. There are companies that put together cultural homestay tours, promising an authentic taste of life on Taquile, but they are too expensive for my budget. I'm also unsure if the extra money actually goes to the residents who open their homes to tourists, so I cobble the trip together myself.

I find a boat headed from Puno to Taquile, with a quick stop at a floating Uros island. It is a queasy, four-hour ride with more passengers than life jackets. When the boat finally docks, the entire island seems to be uphill. The land is lush and green, threaded with stone paths.

About half of the people from the boat are day visitors, and we struggle to hike the demanding hills to the town square. The other boat passengers are Taquileños, who chew the hills with their feet, running ahead.

Though the island has tried to maintain their traditions, there are immediately signs that tourism has affected the tiny community. Some of the markets sell expensive Snickers bars and bottles of Coca-Cola, imported from Puno for the tourists. A small restaurant advertises "American food" along with traditional dishes. Then a small boy follows me, chanting, "Photo, photo." I assume he simply wants to see his image on the digital display, the reason many children along the Inca Trail and in the Amazon approached me, so I stop and take a quick snap. The boy shoves his hand at me.

"Five dollars," he says. "One Abraham Lincoln." I am shocked but also impressed by his knowledge of American currency.

It's tough to shake that moment, though. As someone who has traveled mostly within my own country, I've never considered this ethical situation before. Is it possible to visit a unique place, learn about the culture, and support the economy without changing what makes the place special? I hope so. Because there's a lot that makes this place special.

Among them, the island is home to the most delicate, beautiful handicrafts, recognized by UNESCO as the best in all of South America.

The women of Taquile spin wool, dyed vivid primary colors using local materials. The men are knitters. Boys learn to knit at a young age, around six or seven, and their skill eventually becomes a sign of masculinity. For instance, when a couple intends to marry, the woman takes her love interest's hat and fills it with water. The longer it takes for the water to leak through, the tighter the knit and the better the man.

Once a couple agrees to marry, the woman then cuts off most of her hair to be woven with heavy wool into a thick belt, about eight to ten inches wide. It is long enough to wrap around the man's waist a couple of times.

The wide, thick belt serves two purposes: It is a sign to others that the man is betrothed and is now off the market, kind of like an engagement ring. On a more practical note, the belt also works as a lower back brace—the assumption is that married men carry more burdens than single ones, and they can use the extra support.

Tourists mostly come for the knitted goods, which are displayed around the main plaza. The hats are strung up from ropes like colorful prayer flags.

Scarves and sweaters are folded into neat piles. There is no haggling at this market—everything is a fixed price—and each piece has a tag that says the name of the family that made it, so the money goes directly to them.

I inquire about a homestay inside the craft market, and one man immediately nods, then hands me off to a thin man who doesn't even glance in my direction. He wordlessly leads me through a zigzag of alleyways and streets and passes me off to another friend. The men here all dress the same—black trousers, white shirt, cropped black vest, wide woven belt—and this begins to feel like a blur of the same person. Finally, I meet Thomas.

His face is umber with ruddy spots on his cheeks, and he does not smile. I'm nervous, but I also feel that I'm living under new rules now. I have to squash the anxious part of myself in order to continue moving forward.

When I ask Thomas if I can stay with him for the night, he nods. In exchange for about seventeen dollars, he will provide me with a room for the night, a home-cooked dinner, and breakfast the next day. I follow him about a mile, maybe more, until we reach a property clinging to the side of a mountain.

"Casa de Thomas," he says, and he motions for me to follow him through a low-slung wooden gate.

The house is about the size of a 700-square-foot apartment, built on a plot of gravel and straw. Chickens wobble and cluck, both inside the building and outside.

My room is located in a structure built on stilts adjacent to Thomas's main home. The walls are roughly hewn wood. The ceiling is a blue tarp, pulled tightly and stapled down. There are two simple beds, each topped by five wool blankets. For light, Thomas hands me a small candle in a wooden holder and a box of matches.

There are three other people staying with Thomas that night in a different part of his house. I expected this, knowing that most of the islanders now make a living through such homestays. In the evening, we gather in another room of tarp and wood, where we eat together. Thomas's two young children are also there, but they do not eat—they laugh and play with sticks on the dirt floor. The sun sinks quickly, and though it's only 5 or 6 p.m., it feels like midnight.

Thomas's apple-cheeked wife, Inez, has cooked the food, and I almost laugh when I see what she brings to the table: omelets and French fries, quinoa soup, and bread, the same meal I've had almost every day since I arrived in South America. But the food is rich and hearty and good, and I can't complain. While the wind whips furious outside, I am grateful for my seat at this table and the hot food on my plate.

The moment feels like one from my youth. The sober-faced Thomas, a determined family provider, vaguely resembles my dad. Inez's warmth and willingness to please almost painfully recalls my mom. Whenever I had friends over for dinner as a kid, my mom trotted out pizza and soda and anything to please, as if she could buy my friends' affection with grease and sugar. I was an awkward kid, a total nerd, and she believed that food could fix almost anything, even smooth over my social missteps.

After I finish dinner, I retire to the simple bedroom. It's cold and there's no heat, so I crawl under the thick, wool blankets. It's like the fairy tale of the princess and the pea, if the princess had slept with the pile of mattresses on top of her instead of the other way around.

I long to call home now, simply for a moment of contact in the middle of this vast night, if only someone was there on the other end to answer. I know my dad is at the nursing home this evening, the way he is every night, holding my mom's hand until visiting hours are over and the nurses kick him out.

Though I'm not tired, I blow out the candle and try to fall asleep; then I hear a small noise gradually growing louder. There's a fiesta outside, a loud, raucous party with dancing and singing. The Taquileños must be drunk to be having such fun on a night that is so punishingly cold.

I tried to sleep through a festival a few nights ago in Lima, my last moments with Jason. That sleep was fitful and achy, soaked with tears. The festivities only served as a cruel reminder that other people were happier than me. Tonight, however, I am lulled by the sound of pan flutes and drums as villagers march around the island's winding paths, the slap of sandals against stone.

I still miss Jason, of course. It's the hollow situated just under my rib cage, a place of echoes and rustling leaves, but I'm starting to see how I can live with that feeling there. That ache is becoming a part of me.

Don't Let the Monkeys Get You Down

My next destination is Villa Tunari, and I arrive by minibus, a twelve-hour journey from La Paz, Bolivia, crammed between a bulky man and an old woman who occasionally fondles my nose piercing and laughs. When we reach the tiny jungle town, the driver pauses on a bridge with no shoulder, ushers me out of the bus, and points up the road to a series of small, flat buildings.

I am here to volunteer at a primate sanctuary. The gig is with a non-profit organization that runs a wildlife sanctuary in this remote community that is surrounded by rainforest and overgrown coca fields.

My mother always had a soft heart for monkeys, filling my lunch box with sock-monkey stickers, and she dreamt of seeing one up close, so this feels right: sunshine, an exotic jungle locale, as many bananas as I can eat, and monkeys everywhere.

The people who run the organization are laid-back and noncommittal. When I sent an email last week to ask if I needed to commit to a volunteer date, they responded with a terse message: "No." When I pressed them for more details, they replied with a sheet of frequently asked questions, including a warning about the village's only cash machine. If it is broken, and it often is, the closest ATM is eight hours away. They also recommended bringing enough packaged snacks, medicine, and hygiene products to last the entirety of my stay, since the village markets don't sell much beyond fresh produce and watery beer. I am required to stay a minimum of fourteen days.

I'm anxious, watching the minibus skitter away, and I don't even know if this is the right town. By the time I reach the buildings, I'm sweaty and red-faced but relieved to find it's the correct place. The volunteer coordinator, an Aussie named Noel, takes my passport and ATM cards to store them in a safe.

"You won't need those for a while," she says with a wink.

Noel then takes me to the sanctuary's thrift store, where volunteers rent tattered clothing so our own gear won't be ruined by the work. For just a few dollars, I pick up long-sleeve button-down shirts to keep me covered from the sun; khakis durable enough to resist jungle thorns; knee-high galoshes for hiking through mud and monkey feces.

Wearing somebody else's clothes is transformational, and I wish my mom could see me now. I am no longer the delicate flower who drank martinis in Palm Springs and wore high heels at galas and press events. In these borrowed clothes, I am a new Maggie—a wilder, fiercer version of myself, a rugged me I've never met before.

My room is narrow and made of concrete bricks, painted that particular pink-yellow of cat vomit, topped by a roof ringed with moisture stains and mildew. There is only one door, and it is attached by just one hinge on its lower right side. The bottom of the door has rotted away, leaving a hole shaped like an upside-down U. When I close my door each night, I have to reach through the hole and pull an old tire close to block it, so wild animals won't wander inside. Still, I wake up some mornings and find stray kittens with weepy eyes snuggled up in my piles of clothes. The window has a curtain made of shredded black plastic garbage bags.

My bed has a frame, but the mattress is hard and dusty, stuffed full with some kind of grain. It is filthy enough that I roll out my sleeping bag on top and sleep inside. The combination, however, is surprisingly comfortable.

Noel tells me the area surrounding the animal sanctuary is steeped in the narcotics trade, home to large fields of coca plants. Army helicopters, looking for crops, often circle overhead. It doesn't feel dangerous, though. This is a battle waged on someone else's land, and I have no reason to worry.

I am assigned to work in Monkey Park, an area where about 400 abused and mistreated monkeys, most of them seized from the illegal exotic pet trade, are being reintroduced into the wild. Nearly all of them live in the jungle without cages, but they stick around because the sanctuary provides fresh produce and vitamin-laced porridge twice a day.

My job includes washing fruit and chopping melons for the three daily feedings, filling buckets with bananas, shoveling enormous piles of monkey waste, and cleaning the cages of forty spider monkeys. (Those monkeys are particularly valuable to poachers and traders, so they are the only ones caged and locked away each night.)

Every other day I am also on blanket duty, which means I have to clean the four-by-five-foot pieces of wool that line the cages of the quarantined monkeys. One by one, I scrape feces off each thick blanket and scrub away the stink and disease with a bar of lye and a brush. Then I dunk the sudsy blanket in a bucket of hot water before hanging it on a clothesline in the trees. It is hard work, but it's satisfying. Sometimes I don't even sing or think. I just appreciate the way a pile of dirty fabric transforms into 200 clean blankets, dripping and drying on the lines. The skin on my hands peels raw, and I don't mind at all.

Up until this point, my entire life has been separated from physical labor, other than helping around the house or weeding the occasional garden. My adult years have been spent in classrooms, newsrooms, or the mall, shelving books at a library, making espresso at a coffee shop, or writing at a computer. This work, however, is a revelation—my muscles are sore from shoveling and scrubbing, I pant and wheeze while carrying buckets into the jungle, and I grit my teeth as I chop and prepare food. There is pleasure in finishing each task.

My mother has told me stories about growing up in Germany, where she worked in the fields to provide for her mother, sister, and grandparents, planting seeds, picking potatoes, plucking freshly slaughtered chickens. It makes me feel more connected to her, appreciating her hard work on a level I never experienced before. Her decades of labor meant that I was offered the privilege of avoiding it.

When I finish each shift, I am covered in sweat, mud, and mosquito bites. My fingernails are broken. My cuticles are encrusted with too much dirt to wash away, even when I use a pocketknife to scrape around each crescent. Dinner feels earned.

THERE ARE NO MIRRORS IN THE VOLUNTEER LIVING QUARters, but if there were, I probably wouldn't recognize myself. In the humidity my curly hair quickly goes wild, all tangled and scraggly. There's barely any running water either—the town has been suffering from a drought, so the rare and wonderful shower days are something to be celebrated.

I have been at the sanctuary for one week, and a good portion of every glorious day is spent playing with monkeys. Romeo, a tiny capuchin, often curls around my neck like a living, breathing fur stole. Around ten inches tall, he is smaller than most of the other monkeys, so he fears them. When bigger capuchins come near, Romeo clings to me tightly. He chirps in my ear and tugs at my hair to groom me, as though I'm one of his own.

Anita, a fat capuchin, likes to munch her food and stare at me with her hypnotic dark eyes until I look at her. As soon as I return her gaze, she leaps toward my face, sticks a finger up my nose, then scurries away.

Martina, a barrel-shaped monkey with tufts of dark hair around her jawline like an Amish beard, brings me gifts of rocks. One day when I am sitting, Martina scrambles onto my lap and tugs on my fingers until my hand rests against her belly. I leave it there. A few seconds later, I'm surprised to feel a baby stirring inside her womb. I don't know if this behavior is typical for monkeys, but to me it feels special.

Monkey Park is one small sliver of the sprawling property, which houses more than 700 creatures of all shapes and sizes. Because it is Bolivia's only animal sanctuary, nearly every abused, mistreated, or illegally traded exotic animal in the country is sent here, creating a Noah's Ark–esque collection of pumas, leopards, coatis, bears, birds, and monkeys.

The situation for the already crowded sanctuary is poised to grow even more strained. In July 2009, Bolivia passed a law that declared the use of animals in circuses constituted an act of cruelty, and they passed a ban throughout the country—the first ban on circus animals in the world.

Circus operators were given a year to comply with the law, which meant that they had to get rid of their animals by July 2010. My work at the sanctuary began in August 2010. While I'm there, dozens of animals arrive every day, either turned over by owners or the police.

One monkey, brought in on my second day in the park, had been raised to be a performer. His owner dressed him up in tiny clothes and forced the animal to dance on an electric hot plate. Another monkey had been nearly starved to death by owners who didn't know how to care for him. They kept him in a small box until his howls for help grew too loud and irritating. One of the park's pumas was nearly crippled after jumping through hoops of fire at an illegal circus. His paws were still crispy when he arrived.

TODAY THE SUN IS BRILLIANT AND ONLY SLIGHTLY FILtered by the trees. Green branches and knobby vines weave cathedral-like arches above my head. Tropical birds sing, and monkeys somersault through the air. Then the people with machetes arrive.

The *campesinos*, or farmers, number more than 125 men, women, and even children, all wielding blades. They have been hired by the village government to build a road through the sanctuary, even though the animal refuge has been a part of the local community since 1996. They position themselves along the trail and chop rapidly and haphazardly.

It seems like only seconds before the trees tumble. Every horrifying crackle creates a wide hole in the jungle skyline. It doesn't take long before the tree-lined trails look more like mulch.

An Australian volunteer and I push our way through the campesinos, grabbing monkeys from falling trees. The animals' cries sound similar to those of frightened babies. The howls are haunting and unsettling.

The workers swing their blades toward the monkeys, taunting them. When a mother and baby monkey become trapped in a cage of downed branches, one man steps toward them and brings his machete down like a guillotine, catching the baby on the foot. The older monkey howls as the baby screeches in pain. Another group of men shove a spider monkey into a metal garbage can, then spit on the animal while he cowers. I fight for the animals the best way I know how, by shepherding them to safety, but I sure wish I had a machete of my own.

This new road is supposed to slice directly through the center of the park, displacing hundreds of animals, damaging the delicate jungle ecosystem and destroying the "monkey mirador" area, where violent monkeys are rehabilitated. An official from the village says heavy equipment will show up within a few days to flatten the lush area.

The goal for this road is to create quick, easy access for the local coca farmers to bring their products to bigger communities. Part of this is good. Coca is an important crop in this region of South America, and there are many legitimate uses for it. It's such an important crop that in the 1990s, one out of every eight Bolivians were *cocaleros*, making their living from coca cultivation.

Of course, there are illegal uses for the plant as well. When the leaves are steeped in kerosene and processed with sulfuric acid, the natural crop is turned into cocaine. The government is looking to eradicate the larger farms that exceed what is needed for traditional uses of coca, the places where a plant becomes an illegal drug.

The Bolivians who run the sanctuary gather all the volunteers in the food warehouse to give us an update. They claim the farmers need the road for an easy route to the highway. Trafficking cocaine and making money is the priority to the local village. Not the animals.

Romeo clings to my neck as I pluck another spider monkey baby from a trash bin. More trees fall around us. I have never seen the monkeys so terrified.

A previous attempt was made by the village government to construct a road through the park, but it washed out during a landslide in the rainy season. Managers at the sanctuary expect something similar to happen this time around. No plans have been made for better construction. There is nothing long-sighted about the people here now, chopping down trees.

The distance between home and where I'm standing has never seemed greater. No one tells you this at the start of a journey—that the gap between places can widen so far, it's possible you'll never go back to the place you were.

Three days after the campesinos ravage the jungle, the monkeys remain anxious and unsettled. I don't blame them. The tree line now looks like a smile with several teeth knocked out. Large swaths are missing, and it's more difficult for the monkeys to leap from bough to bough. The trails are obscured by broken branches.

"I don't even know where to begin," says an Australian volunteer.

A young woman named Megan, a former police officer from England, sits on the ground, hugs her knees to her chest, and cries.

"This is the worst thing I've ever seen," she says.

Though the volunteers expected the bulldozers to show up already, they have not. We try to maintain our routine as best as possible, but it's difficult when everyone is anxious. Every morning we expect to find another piece of jungle absent. We barely talk anymore during the daily chores.

I am just about to leave for my own lunch after the mid-morning feeding when a stocky monkey named Reno jumps onto my lap. Reno is the approximate size and shape of a basketball. He's all muscle, but his fur is as soft as a plush toy.

When I stroke his back, he snuggles deep into the crease between my legs and hips. He's not typically a cuddler, so this is a treat. I decide lunch can wait. The sun is shining, and the air smells like fresh rain and papaya. I am content here.

Without warning, Reno hops up and urinates on my thighs. Before that has time to register, Reno hops to the ground, grabs my arms, and sinks his teeth into the flesh of my left hand. It is sudden and shocking, and I inhale sharply but don't make a sound. This isn't like Reno.

The bites become increasingly vicious and quick, aggressive enough to make an audible sound as fang hits bone, and pain dawns on me. I yawp with fear, but I don't know how to defend myself against the unpredictability of a creature I thought I knew. Reno's eyes are wild as he looks up at me, and my thoughts are equally wild. I'm afraid that he might leap onto my face, claw my eyes, rip the hair from my head. He is small but strong.

My long shirtsleeve falls down my arm and covers my skin, and Reno lifts the fabric away, exposing me again. When I try to pull away, he yanks my hand closer, biting down again, gnawing farther up my arm. When blood flows, Reno laps it up like melted ice cream on the side of a cone.

My face is red and hot, and I can't stop myself from screaming.

"The fuck?" I yell.

Just as he eyes my neck and leaps to my shoulder, another volunteer walks into Monkey Park. The sound scares Reno away. I am shaky, and the volunteer puts an arm around my waist and helps me walk down the rocky path toward the main road. He brings me a bottle of water, and then he must get back to work.

I walk by myself from the sanctuary into the small town, about two miles away, the closest place to find help. My wounds are still open and bleeding. I am too stunned to panic.

My first stop is the hospital, but I leave when a receptionist says they cannot promise me clean needles. "Is that okay?" he asks, but I am already walking away. I determine antibiotics are more important than stitches.

On the main street I approach strangers for help, sounding out the word for "pharmacy" in hesitant Spanish.

"Far-mah-SEE-yah?" The blood runs down my hand in hot, slender rivers.

One by one, each person casts a downward glance. Some shrug and walk away. They want nothing to do with the crazy, bleeding lady. Can't say I blame them. The more people reject me, the more agitated I become. Finding a pharmacy is now my mission in life, and I pace the street, stopping everybody I see. I am like the loud and unrelenting beggar on a city sidewalk that can't be avoided.

"Far-mah-SEE-yah?" I say to an old man, who is sweeping the dirt from his dirt patio onto a dirt road. He shakes his head no.

Sobbing, I cry out, "Far-mah-SEE-yah!"

"Ah," the old man says, then he changes the emphasis on the syllables ever so slightly: "Far-MAH-see-yah. Why not say so?"

He ushers me into his unmarked store.

A long glass counter runs the length of the room, crowded with untidy stacks of boxes. The shelves along the wall sag under heavy glass bottles and a rainbow assortment of pills. Near the window, several fat mason jars hold urine-colored fluids and pale spirals of snake bodies.

The old man tosses a stained white coat over his clothes and looks at me expectantly over his half-rimmed spectacles. I hold out my hand, clearly Swiss-cheesed with fang holes.

"*Mono es loco!*" I say in my best Spanish, which is poor Spanish. "Mono … uh, *el* bite-o my *mano.*" I bare my teeth, let out a monkey howl, and pantomime the tearing of flesh.

"*Sí,*" the man agrees, looking me in the eye. "Loco."

His coat swirls as he turns, shimmying around the shelves, grabbing a wide variety of pharmaceuticals. He fans them out on the counter in front of me.

"Which one?" he says.

"*No sé.* Which one for monkey bite?"

He shrugs. I shrug back and point to something with a lot of *z*'s in the name. It sounds important. "*Antibiótico?*" I say.

He shrugs again, then pushes a long package of orange-and-red-striped pills across the counter. The foil is old, peeling from the back of the blister strip.

"Good enough," he says.

It is everything my travel doctor has warned me about—medicine that looks like candy; an open package of pills; a pharmacist in a sketchy store who doesn't speak the same language—so I am skeptical, but I don't have much choice.

This village has five internet cafés and several bars, but only one pharmacy. It would take many hours by bus on dirt roads to reach the next town of any size. In addition, labor protests have shut down the major roads, and it is uncertain if anyone can get through. I am stranded in this town.

The drugs in my pocket still don't change the fact that I need stitches, and the hospital is sketchy. I hurry back to the animal sanctuary and find the staff veterinarian.

The vet is a small, sweaty man with a mild command of English. He tugs a black thread in a zigzag pattern through my skin, ties a knot, and trims the excess. Then he dabs purple fluid on the wound. It looks terrible.

"Better," he says. "Come back if hand becomes pus."

I suppose there's a wildness to everything in our lives; we just don't realize it. I think about how Reno's behavior shifted swiftly, how even the mighty tree line was ravaged in a matter of minutes. It's the same way my mother's disease seemed to strike from nowhere and caught my family by surprise. One day you're surrounded by jungle bliss; the next day the trees fall.

One thing I have trouble admitting, even to myself, is that I'm terrified of what happens if the disease comes for me. I don't want Jason to have to live with the wreckage of my mind. I don't want my family and friends to witness my erasure. Part of the reason I embarked on this trip was to complete my mom's goals, but this is also a battle against the disease itself, cramming myself full of my own memories, hoarding them and holding them tight, before anything is taken.

I know that's not the way things work. The only reliable thing is unpredictability, and diseases strike when you least expect them, as do animals. But I have to try.

That's why I decide to stay at the sanctuary for a few more days. It is an act of courage to be here. It is an act of courage to exist in the world at all.

I tell myself I can handle this, even though it's hard to work when I feel threatened and unsafe. I am hot and hungry and tired of eating bananas. I smell terrible. My body is caked with three days' worth of sweat, dirt, monkey piss. Now blood. Even the monkeys are turning against me. If I hadn't given up so much to be in this place right now, I would buy a ticket and fly home. But what kind of person would I be if I gave up now? The whole reason I wanted to travel was to see what I was made of, to discover how strong I could really be, to live out the dreams of my mother.

I give myself three days before I plan to return to La Paz—cutting short my volunteer stint by just two days—and I'll continue to my mom's next life-list item from there. I'll be at the sanctuary long enough to do more of the work I have loved, long enough to challenge myself, long enough to prove I'm not running away from anything.

Sweetness Remains

———∞∞∞———

A FEW DAYS AFTER RENO'S ATTACK, I TAKE A MINIBUS TO A bigger city and purchase another bus ticket to head to the southern part of the country. I'm aiming for Sucre, a UNESCO World Heritage Site made up of white colonial buildings, magnificent churches, and leafy plazas.

It is dark when the bus finally crawls out of Cochabamba, a city shaped like a soup bowl, where dirt and pollution hang in the air. The elevation coupled with the air quality leaves me breathless, and I'm happy to keep moving.

My large backpack has been stuffed in the luggage compartment under the bus, but I have another, smaller backpack that contains my valuables and a handful of necessities under my seat.

I am dirty. I am worn. I am cold. My hand throbs from monkey bites.

I shove the broken bus window as far shut as it will go. When it won't budge the final inch, I plug an extra pair of socks into the gaping hole. Even with that insulation the air is still frigid. I stuff the earbuds of my iPhone into my ears and crank up George Harrison, which has become the soundtrack for my trip. "My Sweet Lord" provides such tremendous comfort, listening to it becomes its own kind of prayer. Sometimes I wonder if my mom listened to it while she was pregnant, but there's nobody who can answer that question.

I'm wearing my thickest fleece jacket, and I use the other one like a blanket, pulled tight over my body like a mummy wrap. I stretch my hat down over my ears as far as it will go, then wedge a couple of T-shirts between the side of my head and the window. I scrunch my eyes shut and try to sleep, but the vehicle has different plans.

The bus groans up each hill with high-pitched, metallic shrieks, then moans when it reaches the top. This happens often. Bolivia is a hilly country. Once in a while the weak headlights illuminate the landscape, showcasing a world of sheer drop-offs and streets that crumble down the sides of mountains.

Occasionally the driver pulls over to the general vicinity of the side of the road, where he opens the wheezy doors to let more people board the vehicle in exchange for a palmful of coins. Every time I think we can't squeeze another passenger on the bus, we add ten more. The passengers carry burlap sacks—some grain, some potatoes—and pile them high in between the seats. They perch on top of the mountainous lumps like possessive hens.

Then there are the potholes. Nearly every rotation of the tires means another hard thunk of the bus and another thwack of my head against the window.

After an hour, the bus feels like a hostage situation, and I am miserable. I can't recall a life without hairy arms on my neck, bags of bananas on my lap, chaotic bus noise, and strange, fermented smells. I no longer remember what it feels like to sleep without my head smacking a window. Of course, comfort is one of those things that you don't fully appreciate until it's gone.

I knew that backpacking wouldn't be a string of stays at fancy hotels, but somehow I didn't think about hours of numb thighs and teeth-rattling rides along treacherous roads and the feeling that what I am doing is utterly pointless. My mother's disease has brought me here, and for what? She doesn't even know where or who I am.

I could be at home. At home I have a hypoallergenic mattress with a Tempur-Pedic foam top. I have a husband who fits the shape of my body inside his long, warm arms. I have a pillow. And I don't have a hairy stranger in the seat behind me, trying to cop a feel under the guise of dropping his sack of bananas.

I close my eyes, breathe deeply, and tell myself this is all part of the experience. This isn't about staying comfortable. Discomfort was the goal. I just need to change my attitude—one person's bone-jarring bus seat is someone else's vibrating massage chair, after all. Another deep breath. Then I open my eyes.

There, in the seat in front of me, a hefty Bolivian woman hoists her skirt to her waist as she squats to the floor.

I rub my eyes, the way cartoon animals do when they want to wake up. Yep. The woman is still there. Still squatting. How peculiar.

Over the roar of the bus squeaking, the metal heaving, the people snoring, I hear an unmistakable hiss.

"Oh no," I say.

I try to catch the attention of the men seated behind me.

"Oh no."

I point to the woman for anyone who will bother to look.

The bus begins its ascent up another hill.

That's when I remember my backpack.

I reach under the seat for my black bag.

It is slick with wetness and stinks of fresh pee. Thankfully, my backpack has a waterproof lining, so my passport, laptop, and other items inside remain unscathed, even while the backpack itself is soppy with warm fluid. I am too shocked to say anything to the woman, who has settled back into her seat and already appears to be asleep.

After a total of eleven hours, the bus drops us off in the center of Sucre. My muscles ache, my shoulders are bruised, and pins and needles shoot up my legs. My backpack is wet, and I hold it at an arm's length. I'm as grouchy and sour as I've ever been.

The one solace is this place where I've landed, one of the most gorgeous cities I've ever seen. The buildings are sculpted and buttery, like gingerbread slathered in white frosting. It reminds me of the miniature village my mom used to display on the fireplace mantle at Christmastime.

The morning light is golden and diffuse, and the delicate blue of the sky is embroidered with clouds. The lack of congestion and pulsing music gives the town a sensuous, slow-paced feel.

I know I'm supposed to be on a journey for adventure, but I can't find it within me to seek it out today. So I check into a hotel instead of a hostel, even though it's going to cost more money. I just want to unpack.

My room contains a private bathroom, and I fill the tub with water. I scrub myself thoroughly with a rough washcloth and heavily perfumed soap. When I'm clean, I drain the tub and fill it again with water so hot it steams up the entire room, and then I submerge my backpack. As it soaks, the water grows dark, like a sooty tea. I rinse and rinse until the water runs pure.

After I hang the bag to dry, I walk downstairs to the hotel's breakfast buffet. I tear through eggs, fresh fruit, and toast. When the employees aren't looking, I wrap *buñuelos*—fried dough balls—in napkins and slip them into the cargo pockets of my hiking pants. They taste better dipped in honey, but the plain pastry will suffice later today when I'm hungry and alone.

My afternoon is spent walking the historic center of Sucre, where the buildings gleam confection-white, my pockets heavy with Bolivian doughnuts. These pastries are not remarkable, but even so I wish I could share them with my mom, who has developed a fierce craving for sugar over the past couple of years.

Alzheimer's disease tampers with everything inside a body, even the taste buds. One theory is that dementia causes a patient to lose the ability to remember flavor. Others say the distortion of taste buds is a normal side effect of an aging body.

Whatever the cause, the effect is like eating when you have a terrible cold, one of my mom's doctors explained. There's a barrier to the flavors you once knew. When taste is impaired, the only flavors that can break through the barrier are the strongest ones, like salty, fatty, or syrupy sweet.

For my mom, a longtime enthusiast of mint chocolate chip ice cream and red licorice, her tastes always leaned heavily on the sweet side. Now, ten years into dementia, even more so. These days her food pyramid is constructed on a foundation of applesauce and chocolate pudding. When she refuses to eat the overdone vegetables on her dinner plate at the nursing home, a sprinkle of sugar makes them palatable.

I appreciate this. It's the one minor kindness of a horrific disease. When the road stretches long and dark and ragged, it's sweetness that remains at the end of it.

Life Is Worth Celebrating

⸺⧟⧟⧟⸺

There's a TV show I watched in preparation for my trip, a documentary series called *I Shouldn't Be Alive* that features near-death experiences and stories of survival.

"Why are you watching that show again?" Jason would ask. "It's creepy."

"It could save my life," I'd say. "I'm learning what not to do."

I was joking, of course. Though I'd heard plenty of stories about back-packers getting mugged or having their ATM cards stolen, I didn't think my backpacking trip would be a risky endeavor.

My incident with the snake in the rainforest taught me better, and then I was attacked by a monkey in Bolivia. But it's not until I get to Tu-piza that I realize just how easily I could have my very own episode of *I Shouldn't Be Alive*.

Tupiza is Bolivia's version of the Wild West, a small town of red dirt and tumbleweeds, horses and broken liquor bottles. I arrive about a week after leaving the animal sanctuary and cleaning up in Sucre, the stitches from the monkey bite still violet and throbbing.

I book a four-day trek of Salar de Uyuni, Bolivia's great salt flats, with the tour agency that has the best online reviews. This is a place that my mom once showed me either in a book or a magazine, I can't remember anymore. What I do recall is that the photograph of the otherworldly terrain made her gasp as soon as she turned the page and saw it. Blue sky and ground as flat and smooth and white as notebook paper.

"That's salt, Margaret," she said, visibly excited, poking her index finger at the vast expanse of white. It looked like the earth before anything was created for it; a blank slate. "Have you ever seen anything like it?"

I hadn't. But I'm about to.

The tour leaves from Tupiza with a driver, a cook, four other travelers, and myself, taking us through some of the most remote spots of Bolivia before returning to Tupiza.

Right away, the tour goes wrong.

Our mode of transportation is a Land Cruiser that has logged well over 250,000 miles. As it climbs craggy mountain roads, we have one flat tire and some engine problems. We wander the mountain road on foot, taking photos while Carlos, our driver, changes the tire and tinkers under the hood. I don't have a lot of faith in this vehicle.

Though I paid extra for an English-speaking guide, the driver and cook speak only a few words of English. Luckily, one of the tourists is Argentinian, and she offers to translate the driver's words for the rest of us. It is through her that I learn the cook brought only meat-based foods, even though the tour office said it would be no problem that I'm a vegetarian.

We arrive in the rural town of San Antonio de Lipez just as a gray dusk settles. The arid landscape seems barely fit for humans. There are supposedly 250 inhabitants in this place, but I see no farms, no livestock, no people. The mountains are dotted with scrub brushes and crumbling walls.

Our home for the night is a compact structure made of stone and brown clay. The roof is nothing more than a patchy tarp, and snow falls inside the room. There is no heater or running water. When I exhale, my breath forms little clouds. Another tour group joins us—this one with three British men and one British woman, all doing a gap year of travel between high school and college.

I wrap myself in wool blankets, then wiggle into my sleeping bag, cursing the fact that it was made for summer camping. Ali, one of the youngest Brits, dons the sleeping bag he rented from his tour company. The bag is shaped vaguely like a human but comes to a point at each end, giving him the appearance of a giant orange starfish.

"Do you guys think I'm sexy?" he says, posing for us.

"Unbelievably," says Gemma, the British woman. "I can hardly resist you."

We were scheduled to be much farther along the trail by now, but the bad tire and engine problems delayed us a few hours. Also snow is on the horizon, and Carlos says we shouldn't push the vehicle through a storm at night.

Unfortunately, this means we didn't make it to a stop where we could obtain necessary supplies. Instead of dinner, the cook hands over bologna sandwiches and packages of crackers. Gemma pulls a huge bottle of Bolivian whiskey from her backpack. And that's when we are told the bad news.

The British group's guide says the storm is expected to be the worst they've ever seen. With grim faces, the guides give us two options:

1. Ride out the storm in San Antonio de Lipez. The risk, however, is that the storm will linger too long, and we will either freeze to death or run out of food.

2. Find an alternate route through the mountains on rugged, abandoned roads in a vehicle that could potentially break down, far beyond cell phone range or emergency service. We run the risk of getting stranded in the storm, but we'll have a chance of making it to our next stop.

Carlos leaves the decision to us. He disappears with the cook and the other guides outside, where they smoke cigarettes and sip from flasks.

Gemma's whiskey bottle is passed around the table, and each of us takes a hefty nip to stay warm. We breathe on our mittened hands and discuss the pros and cons of each option. Ride out the snowstorm in an uninhabited place with no access to food or heat? Or find an alternate route through the mountains on abandoned roads during a storm in a vehicle that has already proven to be unreliable? Either one is terrible.

We all came here looking for something beautiful and special. Now the landscape is nothing but grim. The frigidness of the air makes me nervous. My bones ache from cold. Will these brown, crumbling walls frame my last memories?

Eventually the discussion takes an even darker turn: with little food left, which one of us should be eaten first?

"I'm out, you guys," I say. "I'm a vegetarian."

"That just means your flesh will be the most tender," Ali jokes. "Like grass-fed beef."

"Maggie it is!" cheers Gemma. "Let's eat Maggie!"

"No!" I laugh, and it is a laugh tinged with fear. We could actually die here. As a tourist, you like to think you're immune to the trouble of the real world, separated from actual hardship and turmoil. It can feel like entering a movie set where everything is picture-perfect and happy endings are guaranteed. The world is not a set, though, and life doesn't play out like a script. Sometimes journeys take a bad turn.

It's what I've seen on every episode of *I Shouldn't Be Alive*. It's never one decision that brings people to the brink of death—it's a series of little, confusing moments that snowball into catastrophe.

That's what I never realized when I was safe at home watching the show: anything can happen at any time. The featured stories aren't about daredevils or extreme risk takers. They are normal people who go for a hike and don't bring enough water. People who take a weekend yachting trip and misread their maps. People just like me and my new friends. Traveling is not a detour from reality. It's simply reality.

By the time the whiskey bottle is empty, we've decided to see what weather conditions are like in the morning before we make a final decision. We sleep, uneasy and shivering on thin mattresses in small rooms.

At 5 a.m., there is a significant layer of snow on the ground. The group gathers at the table and takes a vote. We unanimously decide the better option is to press on, even if it's the last choice we ever make.

All of us huddle together for a picture inside the shelter.

"This will be the photo they'll run on the BBC after our bodies are discovered," Gemma says. We're here in color, breathing and alive, but my mind flashes to the black-and-white photos of doomed explorers in the early 1900s—their faces permanently frozen in smiles, oblivious to what happens next. We have no idea what's ahead either.

My group piles into the tour vehicle, wearing every layer from our backpacks. We spread layers of sleeping bags and blankets over our snuggled bodies. My limbs are too stiff to move.

"*Vamos*," Carlos says, and we set off into the snowy white morning.

The Land Cruiser slides around the road, up and down mountain paths, and everybody in the vehicle is silent. The Argentinian sleeps, while her boyfriend looks worried. I chew my fingernails, a nervous habit I thought I'd long given up.

The realization that I would not have a future was something that came to me when my mom was diagnosed, so this moment is not entirely unexpected. I put myself here on purpose, chasing adventure for the sake of living deliberately and passionately. This is the risk of being an active and living participant in the world. Death happens because life does.

I just thought my moment would come with more activity or splendor, like ice-picking my way up a particularly treacherous part of Mount Everest or BASE jumping off a rocky cliff in Norway. In contrast, this situation couldn't be more passive—I am letting someone drive me directly into the throes of a storm, and there's not a damn thing I can do about it.

In that way, the power of chance is like my mom's disease. There is no reason for the Alzheimer's, and there is nothing to blame. She didn't do anything risky or dangerous; she didn't go looking for a disease. It just happened. Before my family knew what was happening to her, she was already headed downhill into the thick, fierce storm.

I wasn't around when my mom was first diagnosed with her disease; I was working at my first newspaper job and living in Zanesville.

One night my mom was cooking dinner while my dad sat at the kitchen table and watched the news on a countertop television set. My mom had always been a bad cook, but her meals had grown consistently terrible. She made strange stews and pots of spaghetti soup. She used sugar when the dish called for salt. Sometimes she added cracked pepper four, five, maybe ten times. But my dad is a man who cares more about volume than flavor when it comes to his food.

"The craziest thing happened to me today," she said to my father. "Today I forgot how to start the car. Luckily, this nice young man offered to help."

That raised the skin on the back of my dad's neck. The bad cooking was one thing, but she forgot how to start the car?

She elaborated. After she left the hospital for her weekly allergy shot, she sat in the parking lot for several minutes, puzzled, the car's ignition a riddle she couldn't solve. She asked a passerby for help. He turned the key and started the engine, and she drove home.

"Is that just the funniest thing?" she said.

My dad tried to convince my mom to make an appointment with a doctor, but she was stubborn and refused. She accused us of trying to put her in a nursing home, to discard her. Her paranoia worsened, and over the following weeks she became combative.

Since she wouldn't go to the doctor, my dad was determined to bring the doctor to her. He talked to one of the colonels at the air force hospital, who hatched a plan with my mom's regular allergy doctor. The next time she was at the hospital for her weekly visit, they brought in a neurologist. My mom never even realized she was tested—until something from the neurologist arrived in the mail.

The envelope was addressed to her. She opened it. The letter inside said she had failed to answer the simplest questions. She couldn't identify the president of the United States. She couldn't tell time. She didn't know what year it was.

Diagnosis: Alzheimer's disease.

It was the worst way to discover terrible news, and this upended her. As paranoid as she was before, the letter confirmed she had something to be paranoid about: everybody was conspiring against her.

My brother-in-law is the person who finally gave me the news. I knew something was off as soon as he called.

"Something is going on with your mother," he said.

I sat perched on the edge of the futon in my apartment, twisting the phone cord around my finger as he delivered my mom's diagnosis. I struggled to find the words to respond. Then I drove to The Barn, a bar stocked with neon signs, cheap beer, and profoundly lonely people, and I got hammered in the afternoon, because that felt like the only path out of this world where my mom had a disease attached to her.

If I had just not answered the phone, I thought, *Mom would still be well. If I had let the phone ring, everything would still be normal. If I had only let the machine get it.*

On the jukebox I played the U2 song "Sunday Bloody Sunday," belting out the words from my barstool. Then I played it again, until another customer shoved money at the machine to queue up Garth Brooks. I ate a complimentary bowl of peanuts—dinner—and tossed the shells on the floor. I smashed them with my feet every time I stood, a satisfying crunch. I played Erotic Photo Hunt on the game system that was screwed into the bar, finding the five differences between two nearly identical images of naked women, feeding the console dollar after dollar, until the photos softened and the women mushed together and I couldn't spot any differences at all.

Late that night I drove home on the back roads where the only person I could hurt was me. It was January, and everything looked murky and indistinguishable except for the leafless trees that reached over the road with skeletal fingers. I covered one eye with my left hand and steered with my right. All the blurriness that existed around me zoomed into focus, until all I could see were the high beams pointed at the road ahead.

In the Bolivian desert, the snow grows so thick that we can no longer see the other group's Toyota in front of us. Carlos and the cook turn on a Bolivian folk album and keep the same song on repeat. After a while, the rest of us begin to sing along, even though we don't know the words—we're just mimicking the sounds. The music is grating, but singing along keeps me from imagining the truck falling end over end off the side of the mountain, landing upside down in a snowbank, freezing to death.

If I die, I wonder how long it will take for Jason to find out that I'm gone. I sent him several emails before I began this tour with instructions in each message's subject line: "Open this on Day 1," "Open on Day 2," and so forth. He has at least a week of love letters waiting. I wonder what will happen after that last one, what he will think when there are no more messages to open.

The Land Cruiser struggles for traction, and every slide down a hill turns my stomach. The path threatens to crumble every time we slip toward the edge of the mountain. When we can't see a path for all the snow, I wonder how Carlos knows there is actually terra firma beneath us.

The next ten hours are white knuckles and sweaty feet, my nerves tangling into knots. The mountains are snow covered, and our vehicle chews up the gravel. My teeth knock together with cold and fear. When the mountain flattens into an icy desert, our vehicle skates wildly back and forth. It is bleak. The road looks like a Fudgsicle.

At last we arrive at our next stop. Carlos parks in front of a small hostel, similar to the place we just left. This time, however, we have small space heaters. My fingers and toes regain warmth so quickly it hurts. Taking the alternate route meant we missed most of the sights on our itinerary—but we are alive, and the snowstorm is behind us.

Our treat for the night is a dip in the nearby natural hot springs. I submerge myself up to my chin, and my body loosens into the gurgling blue. My chilled bones thaw, a slow and liquid unburdening. I let my neck relax, the back of my head floating on the surface, and I breathe easy and deep. It is almost an hour before I step out of the springs. As soon as I dry off, the tundra air freezes my towel into sculptural shapes, a hardness that mimics the journey we have taken to get here.

The next two days feel like traveling across the moon. In Desierto de Siloli, the lagoons glow with red and green algae, and the bizarre lava formations look like they were stolen from the set of a science fiction movie. Flocks of flamingos along the altiplano turn the sky pink each time they take flight. The ground is white with fields of salt and borax.

On our last night, we stay at a hotel made entirely of salt. The beds are made of rectangular salt blocks, draped with red wool blankets. My friends lick the walls.

In the dim light of that hotel I remove the stitches of the monkey bite, which are pushing out of my skin. I have no scissors, so I snip the top of each black loop with my fingernail clippers, then slide each thread out with tweezers. The flesh around the wound has pulled together and now looks newborn pink. My hand healed when I wasn't even paying attention.

Our final destination is Salar de Uyuni, the largest salt flat on earth, an expanse of 4,086 square miles that stretches down eleven deep layers. The crust also holds about half of the world's lithium reserves.

The desolate landscape deceives the eye. What appears to be one field of snow is actually hard and crunchy salt. You can walk here, but you won't leave any footsteps behind.

Because there is only flat salt and a band of blue sky as far as the eye can see, nothing looks relative in photographs. No mountains to make people seem diminutive, no trees or structures to place anything in perspective. We take photos in which everything is out of proportion—holding hands with dinosaur toys, dancing atop whiskey bottles. At one point the English blokes strip naked and exuberantly leap across the flats—only long enough for some hilarious pictures before they bundle up again in sweaters, scarves, and hats. This is the best day we've had on the trip so far. I'm especially happy knowing the tour will take us back to Tupiza, where I can stay in a warm hostel with a hot shower. I long for this so much, I can already feel the blast of heat on my skin.

It takes many more hours of driving to reach Uyuni, a broken and brown high-altitude town, where the only real attraction is Cementerio de Trenes, a graveyard of abandoned trains. Carlos asks if we want to go there, and all of us say no. It sounds like nothing more than a celebration of the dilapidated and sad. We just want to move through Uyuni as quickly as possible.

Ever since the mining industry failed here, Uyuni has primarily served as a quick bathroom and meal stop for salt-flat tourists like us. It's the gateway of "The Gringo Trail," as we discover the townspeople call it, and it's about four hours from our destination.

It is here, on a dusty and desolate street, where Carlos pulls over to the side of the road. He asks for tips, because the tour is coming to an end. We dutifully hand over a stack of bolivianos. He did get us through a terrible snowstorm, after all, and we are alive.

After he receives the money, Carlos climbs on top of the Land Cruiser. He unleashes the bungees that secured our bags to the roof, and he drops each piece of luggage, one by one, into the dirt. Thunk. Thunk. Thunk.

"No, no, no," I say. I try to toss my backpack on top of the vehicle. Carlos swats the bag away and points a gnarled finger at me.

"No," he growls.

"You're supposed to take us to Tupiza," I say. "That was the deal."

We plead with Carlos, who shakes his head decisively and leaps down from the roof. A cloud of dust rises from the force of his boots on the ground.

When he reaches for the door handle to climb into the driver's seat, the Argentinian tugs on his arm. She stops him long enough to get into a heated argument in rapid Spanish. She points to our bags, then points to the car. After several minutes of fighting, Carlos shrugs his shoulders, hops back into the Land Cruiser, and drives away. He doesn't even look back.

Something about the situation—the cold, the exhaustion, the fact that I am stranded on an anonymous road with nowhere to go—causes me to cackle like a maniac. It burbles up like that hot spring where we soaked a few nights ago, uncorking all the anxiety of this tour.

At least I am alive. It sounds sentimental and soppy, but I have never been so grateful. I have seen the place where mountains crumble under tires, where rugged vehicles are abandoned in the snow, where tourists could very well freeze, where salt forms a vast and grueling landscape, and I emerged on the other side. Getting stranded in Uyuni is a setback, but it's one I can deal with.

"What are we going to do now?" Gemma says.

"Leave," Ali says simply.

My tour group friends and I find a bus station and purchase tickets for later that night—some are headed north, some of us will continue south to

Argentina, most of us will never cross paths again. But tonight we still have a few more hours together.

We spend them at the Cementerio de Trenes, exploring the disrepair. We run on the tracks, and shaggy street dogs run alongside, barking. They want to play. The land around the rotted trains is flat and empty, and the birds overhead make lazy circles. We climb all over the rusted locomotives and bang on the engines, and yawping dogs leap into the trains with us. Then we are listening to the howls, both human and canine, echo through the rusted metal.

Our reverberating laughter sounds vaguely like the chuga-chug of a steam train, and this place of disintegration is once again filled with life. I was wrong when I didn't want to come here earlier. Brokenness makes the cracks that can be filled again. Instead of a disappointment, this graveyard feels like a promise, like potential.

Your Path Might Diverge

———— ⌘ ————

IT'S MY LAST MORNING IN BOLIVIA, AND THE SKY IS DARK, without even a whisper of dawn. The cold is relentless enough to make me dig through my backpack, find my bag of socks (at the bottom, of course), and put a thick sock on each hand like mittens. I quiver each time the wind smacks my cheeks.

The only thing that separates me from Argentina is a bridge. Well, and an office, which is closed. And twenty-seven people standing before me in line, all of whom appear equally anxious to get the hell out of Villazon, Bolivia. But Argentina is close. I know it. And if it weren't 4 a.m., I could even see it.

A couple dozen Bolivian women squat on the sidewalk beneath timid streetlights. Their wool skirts puddle around them on the ground. Each woman is wrapped with several rough, woven blankets, creating the over-all shape of a haystack. Black bowler hats are perched on top of their heads. Shiny black braids hang to their knees.

Across the street is a man, asleep while propped against his wooden fruit cart, his snores echoing on the narrow street. Low-hanging telephone wires crisscross overhead. A pack of wild dogs ambles past.

"Why would the bus drop us off two hours before the border office opens?" says a German traveler, speaking English to his Australian travel companion.

"Because it's Bolivia," his friend replies. "Nothing here makes sense."

After one frustrating month in Bolivia, complete with monkey bites, ice-cold showers, and getting stranded on the salt flats, I have to agree. This morning I am getting out, and I vow to never look back.

At 6 a.m., a man in a uniform unlocks the door of the border office, which is approximately the same size as an office cubicle. Small. About fifty people shove inside at once. The uniformed man is the only person working, and he runs from one window to another—one for Bolivians needing an exit stamp, the other for non-Bolivians needing an exit stamp. Three men in uniforms lean against the wall behind him, drinking steaming cups of tea.

An hour later, when I finally make it to the window, the three men are still standing there. "You like Bolivia?" the man says, nonchalantly, as he flips through my passport and looks over my visa.

"Uh, some bad things happened to me here."

"Very good," he says. He slams a rubber stamp against my passport with a loud *thwack!*

I am ecstatic as I walk toward the simple concrete bridge that forms the border of the two nations. "Argentina, here I come!" I say out loud.

But not so fast. First there is another line for another border office, this time for an Argentinian entry stamp. The line moves quickly, however. There are several men working, all clad in crisp, tidy uniforms. There are distinct lines, with signs explaining entry to Argentina in several languages. The process is straightforward, even when I am pulled aside for a random bag check.

Finally. Argentina. A blazing blue highway sign overhead welcomes: "Bienvenido a la República Argentina."

As I make my way across the bridge and peer over the side, differences between the two countries are already apparent. On the Bolivian side there is a field of stray beer bottles sliding toward the trickling river. Graffiti climbs the sides of structures. Grocery bags flutter against scrub brush, like strange plastic blossoms. The Argentinian side has none of that. No litter. No trash. No spray paint.

At the end of the bridge, a small white sign says "Argentina" in a delicate font, the kind of sign you might find proclaiming "The Smith Family" on the side of a picket fence. It's adorable and strange enough that I snap a photo.

It is an easy walk to La Quiaca, Argentina. I make my way around town on foot in search of two simple things: breakfast and a bank where I can exchange my bolivianos for Argentinian pesos. I walk past an empty park and many closed buildings with shuttered doors. It's rare to see a car drive past. An hour later, my stomach rumbles, I still have no pesos in my purse, and I've walked nearly every street of the small town without finding any food.

An Argentinian tries to help. He says his country enjoys breakfast much later in the day, since they don't eat dinner until 9 or 10 p.m.

"So nobody in this whole town is eating breakfast?"

"Not now," he confirms. "Later."

The same man says the open bank was in Bolivia.

"Not possible," I say. "That would make this the only border town in the whole world without a currency exchange."

"Sí!" the man nods with pride.

I don't believe him, so I walk the streets some more and ask several other residents about the banks. Each person says the same thing: Bolivia.

"ATM?" I am grasping for anything. Any money. Anywhere. Any method. Again, I receive the same word of advice: Bolivia.

I trudge back to the border, back across the bridge, back through the lines of people with sacks of grain. Along the way I pass a white sign that says "Bolivia." It's the same size and shape as the Argentinian sign, but this one is weathered with chipped paint. I don't take a photo.

I FIND A BUS OUT OF TOWN.

When I conjured Argentina in my mind, I saw tango dancers and crowded Buenos Aires streets and steaks as big as platters. I never imagined the landscape of the north, where I am right now: Teal skies that heave with puffy clouds. Arid desert that suddenly buckles and gives way to dramatic expanses of green. Sunlight that dapples the cliffs with pure gold.

I am headed toward Salta, the capital city of this province. For this seven-hour journey, I am pleased to discover Argentinian buses are the opposite of Bolivian buses. The vehicle is well maintained and comfortable, with squishy leather seats, drink holders, and spacious compartments at my feet. The seat reclines so far back, it nearly becomes a bed. Not only is it nicer than business class on a domestic airline, it is nicer than most hostels.

Outside the window, the mountain ranges are wind sculpted, the rock as red as roses, softly folding against each other like ribbon candy. The entire region looks like Sedona, Arizona, with a steroid injection. The roads are smooth, dotted with speed-limit signs and painted lane lines. At home this is standard, but here it feels new and fresh.

For the first time since I started this trip, I have a seat belt, and it makes me feel incredibly spoiled. Who knew a sash of nylon across my lap would bring me such a deep sense of safety? It is a small touch that reminds me of home, security, and protection. I remember the way my mother drove, how her arm instinctively snapped across my chest to squeeze me against the passenger seat every time she was forced to come to a quick stop.

"I have never been so happy for laws," I write in my journal.

I FOLLOW A TRAIL OF WINERIES FROM SALTA TO CAFAYATE, where the sandy soil and mountain air work together to create torrontés, a magical white wine varietal that doesn't exist anywhere else in the world.

I am traveling now with Barbara, a friend from home. We're the same age, in the same place, both making treks around the world, but we're at different places in our lives. The same month I got married, Barbara divorced a man with whom she spent eleven years, a man who also happens to be a good friend of mine. While I am hoping to do some soul-searching on this trip and to make some connections within myself, Barbara is connecting with other people. Specifically, men. But I don't realize this until we begin traveling together.

I have this hypothesis about breakups: after a long-term relationship dissolves, a person regresses to the age they were when the relationship began. Barbara was with her husband for eleven years, ever since they met in college, which turns back her relationship clock to age eighteen.

That's exactly how she appears to me now, and it's nothing like the Barbara I knew before. Physically she has changed, letting her blonde bob grow long and unruly, and her body is thinner. But the most drastic changes are on an emotional level. She is more carefree, which is something I admire, though she's becoming increasingly reckless.

She's eager to hitchhike and collect wild stories. One night she follows a German backpacker to a seedy part of town that we've been warned about, just to flirt with him and score a free meal. Another night she has sex with a Kiwi on the floor of our hostel bathroom.

She's also a thoughtful, intuitive friend, and I cling to her. Part of it is that she can speak a meager amount of Spanish, which is helpful. Part of it is that I have called home again, and my mother is more lost and confused than ever. Her body has developed infections, but she no longer has the ability to communicate her pain. The nurses discover that my mom has been suffering urinary tract problems and earaches, and it's possible they have been blazing for weeks. Her body is breaking down one piece at a time, and I can't do anything about it. Things seem to be crashing down, and I ache for the comfort of the known, even if it's the remains of a friendship.

Together Barbara and I decide to head to Argentina's wine country, a place that appears to offer both tranquility and a party scene.

After the harsh conditions of Bolivia, even the simplest pleasures in Argentina feel downright indulgent. In Cafayate, Barbara and I leisurely bike to local bodegas and stuff ourselves on pumpkin empanadas, creamy leek stews, and wine gelato. We walk a town square where women smile and old men tip their hats. After a few days of bliss, I am relaxed and ready for my first CouchSurfing experience.

CouchSurfing is a website that began in the early 2000s as a way to connect travelers all over the world with hosts, who volunteer lodging in their own home. Hosts cannot charge for their services, which means CouchSurfing is friendly to my meager backpacking budget—but it's also part of a bigger, more lovey-dovey concept. The idea is to find new friends, personalize your travel experience, and learn about a culture from the people who live it. It's about making connections worldwide.

To ensure that nobody is a serial killer, both the host and the traveler create profiles and leave public feedback about each other after a meet-up occurs. So a traveler can peruse host reviews, just like they would with a restaurant or hotel. Likewise, the hosts know that they're not opening their doors for an ax murderer. Both parties agree to the meet-up before any detailed information is exchanged.

Barbara spends a week corresponding with one particular CouchSurfing host, a young American who schlepped her husband and three children through South America before settling in Argentina.

"Her name is Willow, and she is super awesome," Barbara says. "She's a writer, her husband is a film director, and they met when they were doing movie stunts in California. She's into gymnastics, Hula-Hooping, and fire dancing, and she loves red wine, dark chocolate, and books by the Brontë sisters. And they're both trapeze artists and vegetarians."

"Wow. This chick sounds cool."

"It gets better," Barbara says. "They live in a huge, three-bedroom farmhouse that they renovated. And they have dogs and a pool. And bathtubs. The kicker is that they're just outside of Mendoza, which is wine country. And, bonus: they said we can stay as long as we want. Who knows? This might actually be a vacation."

Willow sends directions to her house, but she also asks for a few host gifts—chocolate, a bottle of wine, plus toys for her kids—in exchange for providing shelter. Barbara agrees and confirms our arrival date and time.

We arrive in Mendoza by bus several hours later, bags of gifts in tow, but there is no sign of Willow at the station.

"Weird," Barbara says, rereading her email from Willow. "I didn't notice this until now, but this says we need to get on another bus."

"I thought you said she lives in Mendoza."

"Well, outskirts of Mendoza. Same thing."

I'm annoyed, but there's no reason to vent right now. It's not Barbara's fault we're zigzagging all over Argentina. We buy tickets for San Rafael, as instructed.

Three hours later, we are still on a bus, far outside of wine country. This ride is quiet. I just want to reach our destination, and I have nothing to say to Barbara.

From San Rafael, we catch another bus.

Since Willow isn't around for me to blame, my frustration is unleashed on Barbara. "Where the hell does she live? Chile?" I snap.

"Next time you find the CouchSurfer!" she snaps back.

"I will," I say. "If I'd found the CouchSurfer, we'd be in Mendoza drinking wine right now."

The bus driver looks in the rear-view mirror and smiles. He must be used to taking foreigners to this place, because he doesn't even ask for our destination. He simply pulls to a stop in front of a ramshackle wooden building, then points to Barbara and me.

"Us?" I point to my chest.

"Sí," he nods.

Barbara and I reluctantly step off the bus. The building looks less like a farmhouse than a crime scene. It is encircled by mud, withered crops, and rotting fence posts. And the bus that's driving away is the last of the day.

"Well, it's not exactly wine country...," Barbara says, letting her sentence trail off into the wasteland that surrounds us.

"More like swine country."

Just then a pack of dogs jumps out the front window of the house and tears through the mud and into the gravel road. Their fur is thin, showing raw patches of pink skin. They surround out feet and nip at the air around us.

"Oh, good," I say. "I haven't had mange yet."

Barbara grimaces and pulls away from the dogs. She has been battling ringworm, picked up a couple of countries ago from a stray kitten.

We walk to the house, because there is nowhere else to go. Along the way, we approach a scrap of brown grass where a woman is facedown on a towel. Barbara clears her throat, but the woman doesn't move.

"Is she dead?" I nudge her with my foot.

The woman turns over, props herself on one elbow, and squints at us. "Oh, hey," she says; then she turns back to her towel. Her bikini top slides off.

She is facedown again.

"Wait! Are you Willow?"

At this, she sits up and blinks. She's not self-conscious about her toplessness at all. "No. Duh. I'm Ashley," she says.

"Ashley? Who's Ashley?" I ask.

"I'm ... you know," she sighs. This clearly requires a lot of effort. She sighs one more time for good measure. "The babysitter."

Ashley the Babysitter sits all the way up and spreads her legs, then rubs at the spot where her bikini bottom meets her crotch.

"Look," she says, tugging the bikini fabric from her skin. "I had a big cyst removed from my labia yesterday. And now it's not lookin' too good ... Geez, what's wrong with me?" Ashley abruptly jumps off the towel. "I'm so freaking rude!"

With that, she runs into the house. A few seconds later she returns. "Here," she says and she shoves her fist toward me. "A joint."

THE CHILDREN ARRIVE WITH AS MUCH SUBTLETY AS A gunshot. Evie, Reese, and Liam are a tiny barbaric threesome, like the lost boys in *Peter Pan*. I have no idea where they've been, but once they enter the property, they tumble, pinch, punch, yell, and yawp, kicking up dust, tufts of grass, and stray gum wrappers.

"I'm Reese!" shouts the middle child, who has branches sticking out of her blonde hair like antlers. She is nine years old. "But I demand you call me Saffron Moonblood!"

When I say I'd rather not, she kicks me in the knee.

Evie, age twelve, points to the living room drapes. Five-year-old Liam is already tangled in the fabric near the curtain rod.

"Are you allowed to be doing that?" I say.

All three children reply in unison, "Yes!"

Of course they are. They are allowed to do anything they want, because Willow isn't there. Her husband isn't there either. And we have no idea when either of them will return. Whenever Barbara and I ask Ashley about it, she waves her hand around and says, "Oh, you know." Turns out she isn't as much of a babysitter as a friend of a friend who showed up one day with a bag of weed.

Two hours later Barbara finds a note, written by Willow on a piece of cardboard. It says that she and her husband heard about a film shoot—the landscape surrounding Mendoza is often used as a low-budget Grand Canyon for movies and TV shows—and they will be gone for several days. But they have left us a couple of rules for running the household: Feed the kids. If they want to go to school, they can. If not, hey, don't force them.

Feeding the children is a challenge. The house has little food, the propane tank for the stove is empty, we are many miles from town, and the final bus for the day has long gone. Plus Ashley the Babysitter is stoned and staring at her labia.

"It's fine," says Liam. "I know how to make a fire."

"Seriously? Because I don't," I say.

The boy has clearly done this before. He heaves logs into a squat little stove in the living room. He plucks a match from a tattered cardboard book and gets the fire going. I set a pot of water on the surface. While we wait for it to boil, Liam uses a tiny ax and some fallen branches to build a small bonfire in the front yard. He surrounds it with a ring of stones.

"Hey, Liam, do you usually have more food around here?" I ask, while I help the boy pull together the pile of wood.

"Nah. Not really. Only when my mom asks CouchSurfers to bring some stuff," he says. "Sometimes I go to the next farm, over there, and I ask them for food, and they give us stuff from their gardens. They're real nice."

My mind wanders back to my elementary school years in Ohio, when my parents struggled to put food on the table. My dad was too proud to let us accept any assistance, like food stamps or the free school-lunch program, so it was a burden to feed three kids. Meat was a novelty. But my dad planted a garden in our backyard, which gave us an abundance of vegetables. My mom bulked up our meals using this fresh produce, so our spaghetti was fat with zucchini and cauliflower, casseroles were layered with carrots and squash, and our salads overflowed with radishes, sugar snap peas, and tomatoes. In the winter we ate all the same things—just canned versions of them. It took many years for me to discover how poor we were back then, because I never went to bed hungry. My mom made sure of it.

Water comes to a boil on the stove. Barbara stirs a package of dry pasta into the pot, and I scrounge up a tin of tomatoes and enough condiments to combine for a decent sauce. I plop the pasta onto plates, and the kids tear into their food like lions descending on a fresh carcass.

"Look at my full belly!" Liam says, pulling up his shirt and pushing his stomach out as far as it will stretch.

"When you are in America, do you eat peanut butter?" Saffron Moonblood says.

"Of course! I love peanut butter," I say. "That's what I miss the most." Evie nods.

"You know what I miss?" Liam says. "Toothbrushes."

"Yeah, remember how in California we would brush our teeth? Every night?" says Saffron Moonblood, almost as if she didn't believe it herself. All the children nod.

After dinner, we gather around the bonfire outside and look at the stars. Barbara shows the kids how to find the Southern Cross. When I shiver from the cold air, Liam uses a metal shovel to scoop hot embers and make a pile of them under my plastic lawn chair.

"Now you're toasty warm," he says. He scrunches his nose and gives me a crooked smile. It is sweet, if unsettling, to see such a young child playing with fire. I also feel slightly askew, then realize my seat is melting. I scooch the chair back until the plastic cools and becomes solid again.

Later Barbara and I sit on the couch in the living room with Evie and Liam in a pile on top of us. Ashley the Babysitter is passed out in the master bedroom, snoring loudly. Saffron Moonblood pulls boxes from the closet and finally emerges with a few pieces of old newspaper—a couple of advertisements and the obituary section.

"Can you read to us?" she says, climbing on top of my lap.

"Of course, sweetheart," I say, using my hand to brush the leaves and sticks from her hair. Again, I feel like something is melting.

Back in California, Jason and I have often talked about having children, but I do so in abstract terms. He'd like a child. I am less sure.

I've told Jason that I want to wait because a baby will chain me to a life of sticky playdates and diaper duty.

"Someday," I've said.

What I've never said out loud is that I'm afraid. Every time I misplace my keys or leave my purse in the car, I text my sister in a panic, believing I'm in the early stages of Alzheimer's myself. Shortly after my mom's diagnosis, my dad tried to comfort me on the phone: "By the time you're old enough to worry about it, there will be a cure for this disease," he said. "There might not be hope for your mom, but there's hope for you." Almost a decade later, we are no closer to a cure or a way to prevent this thing. But I am closer to an age where I need to make a decision.

I don't want to be a parent if I can't be fully present and mentally aware. I don't want my child to watch me disintegrate the way I witnessed my mom's decay. And I don't want to pass the disease on. Parenthood is an enormous risk.

However, the choice feels simple in this living room, where the wallpaper peels and the roof sags with mold. I wonder what I am waiting for. I wonder if not taking a chance is, in fact, the bigger risk.

"Barbara, if we don't leave tomorrow, we can't get out until Monday because the bus doesn't run on the weekend. So I think we should—"

"Why would we leave?" she interrupts.

"Uh, because this place is filthy. The toilet doesn't work. There's no food. We are far from civilization. And we're stuck with one weirdo girl. This is like the beginning of a very scary movie."

"It's fun. Relax. You're too high-maintenance."

"I don't think food is high-maintenance."

"Our hosts have been kind enough to open their house to us—"

"What hosts? They didn't even bother to stick around. Oh, and they left three kids here," I say. "I am not a parent, Barbara. I have no idea what I'm doing, except trying to keep three kids fed and making sure the house doesn't burn down."

"We're CouchSurfers. We can't be picky."

"Exactly. We're CouchSurfers. Not babysitters."

My heart breaks for the children. They need structure. They need books and toys. They need to go to school. At the very least, they need to have a responsible adult around to make sure Liam doesn't fall off the roof.

Barbara, on the other hand, admires their blithe, casual lifestyle. She believes important skills are learned outside of the classroom, and these kids are picking up things that will prove valuable later in life. They know how to create their own fun without relying on TV, video games, or other manufactured forms of entertainment. They know how to climb trees and fend for themselves, and they are quick to pick up Spanish. And they are practically welded to each other, so tight is their bond, since they have no one else.

"At least we're learning about the culture." Barbara shrugs.

"How are we learning about culture when we're in a farmhouse, babysitting three American children?"

A voice from the bedroom interrupts our bickering.

"You guys," Ashley the Babysitter yells. "I think my cyst is coming back. Could one of you come look?"

With this, Barbara finally agrees that our time in Argentina might be better spent elsewhere. She and I leave the next morning, headed for the city of Mendoza. When I walk toward the dirt road, Liam clings to my leg. I shake him free, then crouch down to look at him face-to-face. I swipe a lock of blond hair from his eyes.

"I'll miss you, buddy."

"Not as much as I'll miss you," he says.

I have to keep moving before he sees me cry.

IF YOU TASTE SOMETHING DELICIOUS IN ARGENTINA—
creamy gelato, crackly *pan de campo* country bread, vibrant popsicles infused
with lemon verbena—chances are it emerged from Mendoza's rich food
culture. The region is the nation's leading producer of garlic and tomatoes,
which grow as plump as red delicious apples. The empanadas are the flakiest
in the whole country, and the olive oil tastes just like fatty sunshine. Or-
chards line the rolling hillsides.

Of course, there's also the wine. With the largest acreage of malbec
vines in the world, Mendoza is particularly known for this silky, mineral-rich
wine, produced from a thin-skinned grape that needs a lot of sun and heat
to mature.

Although this is an extremely dry desert region, Mendoza has an elaborate artificial irrigation system, diverting melted snow from the nearby Andes into reservoirs, which allows for extensive greenery. That includes the
picturesque, tree-lined city avenues, as well as the more than 800 bodegas
that produce most of Argentina's wines.

Barbara wants to get some exercise, and I want to sample some of the
local products. She and I compromise with a bodega bike ride, which pairs
cycling—a traditionally healthy activity—with binge drinking.

We find a rental place, where we get one map and two wobbly red bikes.
Mine doesn't have brakes, but it does have a bell. The owner, Mr. Hugo,
also promises us unlimited free wine when we return. A backpacker's dream
come true.

Our plan is to ride to the farthest bodega on our map, then work our way
back toward Mr. Hugo's, hitting several more bodegas along the way. That
way, we will only have a short distance to ride when we are most intoxicated.
It is a good plan, but it is quickly derailed.

Barbara and I pedal past a winery that we can easily see from the gravel road. It looks deliciously inviting—a sunny patio, an arch of flowering purple vines, and a big, whitewashed sign that says, "Sip back and relax."

"Should we stop here before we go on?" I say.

"Might as well," Barbara agrees. "We're here anyway."

In exchange for a few pesos, the winemaker himself bends toward us, showcasing one aromatic wine after another. My first sip of malbec is crushed velvet in a glass. The taste is jubilantly spicy and snappy—ripe berries with a twist of black pepper.

"To backpacking!" Barbara says.

"To Mendoza!" I say.

Just then, a cute boy walks toward us, a girl on each arm.

"Ari?" Barbara says.

Ari is a nineteen-year-old whom Barbara slept with back in Bolivia. He doesn't look at Barbara, but his features twist into an uneasy expression.

"Ari. Over here!" Barbara waves her hands in the air. Ari abruptly pulls away from his female companions and turns the other direction.

"I forgot something," I hear him say. "Come on, let's go."

He jumps onto his bicycle, which is parked on the bike rack next to ours.

"Wait!" Barbara runs to her bike too.

"Where are you going?" I yell after her.

We still have two almost-full glasses of perfectly good wine. Why should we have to sacrifice those?

Barbara is already on the street, pumping the pedals hard to catch up with Ari. She doesn't care that he's accompanied by other women—and he seemed happy about it too. I toss my wine back like a shot, then do the same with Barbara's glass. I straddle the wobbly bike and start after her. I pedal until my feet are as dizzy as my brain. Are my legs always this drunk?

"Heeeey! Don't leave without me!" I holler at Barbara, who is now a half mile ahead of me. Her blonde head looks blurry.

Ari gains some distance on her and maneuvers a quick turn. Barbara stops at an intersection, unsure of which way he has turned. I catch up a few minutes later and slow my bike down by crashing into a tree.

We stand on the shoulder of a gravel road, which stretches so far into the distance it looks like it's headed nowhere at all. Barbara straddles her bike. Mine is a heap of metal at my feet.

"I know that was him," she says.

"You don't need him," I say. "He's just some silly nineteen-year-old."

"But I liked him."

"I know. But he's a boy. A child. Seriously, he's not mature enough to handle you."

"You know what I'm going to do?" Barbara says. "I'm going to go back to the hostel tonight and send him a really bitchy email."

"Just let it go. It was a fling. He doesn't want a relationship."

"I don't want a relationship either," she says. She pauses, then sniffs. "It's just—well, I guess I just wanted him to like me back."

I step over my bike and give Barbara a hug. "He did," I assure her.

I don't know if he did, but it's something she needed to hear. We sprawl in the grass off the side of the road, and I hold my friend. We are sad, and we are drunk, and the only thing I can do is sit in my friend's pain with her.

That evening we decide to split up for a while, and we don't acknowledge the ways travel can strain a relationship. Instead, we chalk it up to our dramatically different to-do lists.

I don't know enough about marriage yet to understand how Barbara is struggling to navigate life again as a single woman. On the flip side, Barbara has two young, healthy parents and can't fathom how it feels to have a mom die in slow motion.

I'm headed toward the bustle and energy of Buenos Aires and everything that the city will bring. Meanwhile, Barbara has her eye on the ski resorts of Bariloche, which happens to parallel the trail of her nineteen-year-old flame. We agree to stay in touch over Facebook and meet up again before the end of the month in the capital city.

Our final meal together is a shared platter of pasta in the town square, Plaza Independencia. We each lift a wineglass, and we toast to our separate roads.

Scatter Your Heart
Wherever You Go

—⚬⚬⚬—

People tell me I will die in Buenos Aires.

It began at the job I left behind, where my former colleagues started a death pool, placing bets on where I will meet my demise. The number-one choice was Buenos Aires, though nobody could provide a specific reason.

This didn't have much of an impact back in California. It was a dark joke, but I laughed. Now approaching Buenos Aires, I am both alarmed and superstitious. Compounding that are the stories gleaned from other backpackers in South America, who frighten me with tales of bag slashings, purse snatchings, and muggings gone wrong. Almost everyone has a friend of a friend who was kidnapped.

It makes me paranoid. As soon as my bus hits the city limits, I am on guard, darting my eyes up, down, and sideways, observing every potential thief and murderer. I don't like to be this way—it is exhausting to travel while afraid—but I don't know how to stop it either.

I check into a hostel on Avenida de Mayo, the leafy, elegant heart of the Buenos Aires financial district. The owner gives me a map of local neighbor-

hoods, a list of things to do, and some suggested attractions. Then he turns
serious, his thin lips set in a long dash across his face, and he runs a hand
through this hair.

"Be careful out there," he says. "Not safe for a girl alone."

With that warning clanging around in my head, the streets seem to
transform as I walk them. I stand and watch a cook through the window of
the restaurant on the corner. He slaps a sheet of pasta on a table and attacks it
with a knife, and this innocuous act makes me jump. Every alley looks scar-
ier and more shadowy than the last. Dramatic architecture appears to lean
menacingly over the sidewalks. A man on a crowded street grabs a fistful of
my ass when I pass by.

I don't want to eye every stranger as a potential attacker, but I'm alone
and the city is bigger than anything I've encountered on my own before. I
am smart about how I travel through it, but I look like a tourist—my face
betrays me with a wide-eyed look of half confusion, half discovery—and I
am treated as such. On the cramped subway, commuters packed hipbone
to hipbone, I feel someone unzip the pocket on my hiking pants and shove
a hand inside. There are limbs everywhere—it's like riding the train with
the multi-armed Hindu goddess Kali—and I can't determine where the
hand is attached. I clutch my small bag with my passport and wallet close
to my chest and silently applaud myself for not keeping anything in my
pockets.

The city makes me feel brand-new to the world, but not in a good way.
It's like I'm an infant attempting things for the first time, and it takes too
long to do even the simplest tasks. When I try to mail a package home to
my husband, I am at the post office for six hours before the box is finally
stamped and thrown into a pile with other international mail. It takes another hour to find a Laundromat. When I do, I hand over all my clothes, for-
getting that I will still need something to wear later that night and the next
day too. This is my third month on the road, and I've apparently forgotten
how laundry works.

I go shopping and I don't know how to say no when a slim saleswoman
joins me in the dressing room and squeezes me into the wrong size jeans. The

button sinks into my skin, and the waist leaves an angry, red ring around my middle. I can't breathe, and I point to my rear and explain, "*Grande.*" I am tall, and my body is generous, and I'm angry with the space I take up; I'm mad I can be so large and still vulnerable. I wish my body were something else entirely.

Mom was the same way. Around the time I hit junior high, our house became a world of weekly weigh-ins, diet gum, and Tab. I don't recall my mom eating bread, only thin Wasa crackers at thirty-five calories each. Sometimes she binged on candy or ice cream, then berated herself. She spent years hungry, skipping breakfast and eating only the tiniest of lunches. She was consumed by her own consumption, and when she looked in the mirror, she punched her hips with dissatisfied fists, as though she could smash her silhouette into a smaller shape.

The saleslady pulls another pair from the rack, equally tight but with more rhinestones around the pocket. She shoehorns me into them, wedging my thighs into the denim, and when she bends close to me, her elaborately teased hair smells like cigarettes and powder. When she nods with satisfaction, I give up and buy the jeans. Maybe this is who I am in Argentina, the kind of person who wears painted-on jeans bedazzled in bling. Maybe they will help me slip through the streets unnoticed.

Wearing my jeans and walking past a gun store downtown, I step inside without even making the conscious decision to do so. I don't want a gun, of course. It's irresponsible and would make for some seriously impractical backpacking gear. But I do want the feeling of added protection, something small that I can keep close at hand.

The walls of the shop are lined with glass cases that run ceiling to floor. They contain enough firearms to supply every actor in a Rambo movie. Including extras. Several weapons under the front counter look suspiciously like grenades.

It is a small, cramped shop, so I don't get far before a few employees descend and ask if I need help. At least, I think that's what they've said.

After the *farmacia* debacle in Bolivia, I now possess a Spanish-language guide. But it only includes basic sentences like "Where is the bathroom?"

"Do you take travelers checks?" and "Those drugs aren't mine." I do not possess any real Spanish conversational skills.

"*Hola! No hablo mucho español*," I apologize. I furiously flip through the guide. Unfortunately, none of the words I need are listed.

"*Donde puedo comprar* … pepper spray, *por favor?*"

The employees stare. Nobody breathes a word.

"Er, spray *de pimiento?*" I try again.

Nothing.

It is time to pull out all the stops. It's time for charades.

I give an Oscar-worthy performance: First I play the role of an innocent woman walking down the street. Then I hop a few steps to my right and act out the character of a brutal attacker who punches the woman in the face. Just as the attacker is about to make off with her valuables, our heroine pulls pepper spray from her pocket and shoots him in the eye, sending him kicking and screaming to the floor.

I look up from where I am now crumpled on the dirty, stained tile. My wild charade has drawn a crowd of customers. I had no idea so many people would be shopping for guns on a weekday afternoon. I try again, "Spray de pimiento?"

I'm out of breath and slick with sweat. I mime spray in my eyes and say, "Psssst."

"Ah," someone finally says, and a few other people nod with recognition and exchange quick words in Spanish. A man tugs on the sleeve of an employee, says a few sentences, and motions to me.

One of the gun-shop employees ducks behind a curtain. When she returns, she hands over a plastic-wrapped package of pepper spray.

"Mace," she says.

MY ROOM AT THE HOSTEL IS LAVENDER, AND THE WINDOW opens to a side street off Avenida de Mayo. I've been here more than two weeks. I haven't needed to use my mace, nor have I even reached for it. I keep it tucked into a secret pocket in my backpack, which I keep in the room most days.

The city buildings now appear whimsical and inviting. Most are stately and gray, a fusion of Baroque, Beaux Arts, and Art Nouveau styles. The cool stone is detailed with elaborate carved flowers and vines, gargoyles and fantastical creatures, an architectural landscape that rivals nature.

Across the street is Palacio Barolo, once the tallest building in all of South America, now home to Spanish language schools, a dry cleaner, and some attorneys. The architect was inspired by Dante's *Divine Comedy*, and he integrated artwork, tile, and other design elements into the building to create distinct layers of hell, purgatory, and paradise. The building is one hundred meters high, one for each of the poem's cantos, and the twenty-two floors represent twenty-two stanzas. On a clear day, they say you can see all the way to Uruguay from one of the tiny cupola windows, though when I climb to the top, I can't see beyond the wide, sparkling expanse of the city. I don't want to anyway.

I take the English-language tour of Palacio Barolo twice. Then I return a few more times just to sit in hell, which is lined with attorney offices, and read books. It's quieter than my hostel, and I am comfortable among the Latin inscriptions, a smattering of dragon sculptures, and the fire-patterned floor.

Argentina is a country of immigrants, and the European influence is evident throughout the capital city, not just in Palacio Barolo. Many afternoons I duck into cafés to drink fizzy mineral water with an espresso or enjoy a cup of gelato, and everything about it reminds me of my mom and her Euro elegance.

Before my mom became ill, her face was chiseled and fine, like the stone of the Italianate architecture. She also had grand taste despite our budget lifestyle. When given the option, she preferred sparkling water to still, cashmere to cotton, bitter dark chocolate to anything milky. Her German accent, which I didn't realize was thick until I grew up and moved away for a while, confused my friends and prompted laughter. It was strange because I loved the way she spoke. Her voice sounded urgent and melodic at once, as if she were running to get in front of each word.

She was a woman out of place, not suited for our small town in Ohio. Even though I loved her, as a child I was embarrassed by her foreignness. In a cafeteria full of bologna sandwiches, I carried a lunch box packed with liverwurst. A kid on my block said our house was the only one that smelled like sauerkraut. She didn't wear jeans or have feathered hair, not like my friends' moms; she never looked casual. And here's the tragedy of it all: now that I'm mature enough to appreciate her specialness, the disease has taken everything that made her unique.

She would have loved this city.

At night I stroll through the Palermo neighborhood, a trendy barrio with cobblestone streets, tiny cafés, art galleries, and fashion boutiques. There is energy here, and it's palpable, even from my outsider's perspective. Every street feels like it unravels just for me, and I'm eager to be part of the throngs of people, the restaurants that don't fill until midnight, the clubs that pulse until 6 a.m.

I try on lacy dresses and find the European candies of my childhood. I settle onto a concrete bench in the park and watch young couples woozy with new love and old couples still in love. They hold hands and neck (people still neck?) and trade sips of hot maté served in dried gourds.

I marvel at the people who pass by me—the people who didn't exist in my world until that shared moment on the sidewalk. High-heeled women with swishy, camel-colored hair, old ladies with bright lipstick, elderly men who meet my gaze and wink. A man plays the accordion on the street, and the wheezy song sounds like something I might have once known, maybe something from one of my mom's records. A woman walks past and compliments me on my jeans, the tight denim sausages with rhinestoned designs on the pockets.

Tonight I go out to La Bomba de Tiempo, an improvisational percussion party held every week in a venue that looks like an industrial warehouse. The room is packed with hundreds of sweaty people, bodies moving together, all dancing to the same tune. Every strike of a *tumbadora* matches the thump of my pulse. I have always been a self-conscious dancer, but not tonight. Tonight the music is so loud that it feels like it's coming from inside me. Tonight I dance almost until the sun comes up, sometimes caught in a wave of motion so strong, I'm almost hanging on for dear life. There are masses of people around me, and I don't know them, but our relationship is reciprocal—we feed off the energy of each other. I leave exhilarated, smiling, feeling nostalgic for Buenos Aires before I even leave.

I've been in this city for more than two weeks, and I know it's time for me to move on, but whenever I consider leaving, I am filled with a desperate sense of longing. I'm tempted to call off the remainder of my trip to stay in Buenos Aires. I can't pinpoint the source of that desire, though—I don't know if this is where I could really stay or if this is just a passing moment of comfort. Either way, I wish I could sustain it. This is as satisfied as I've been in a long time.

It makes me wonder about the nature of home, what it means to feel so comfortable in a place where I have no roots, no right to stay, and no reason to belong.

They say home is where the heart is. But there's no easy idiom to apply to my situation: If I am scattering tiny pieces of my heart all over the globe, what does that mean for my sense of home? How will I ever belong anywhere when parts of me are forever in exile? My heart is in a condo in California, nuzzling the warm crook of my husband's neck. My heart is in a nursing home in Ohio, tucked inside my mom's sterile white bed. Now my heart is here, in a city that is bright and complex and as sweet as nectar, a city that I love in part because I first feared it.

THERE'S JUST ONE MORE THING BEFORE I GO: I REMEMBER flipping TV channels with my mom and how she was awed by the athleticism of soccer, the only sport besides Olympic figure skating that she ever paused to watch. And that's why I have to attend a Boca Junior football game.

The reputation of Argentinian football matches is that they are rowdy and wild, and it can be dangerous for people unfamiliar with the stadium, the environment, and etiquette of the fans. This is why tourists are told that the safest way to experience the games is with an escorted group. I book a tour with my new friend from the hostel, Jeff, an American who is all dimples and a toothpaste-commercial smile.

This is one of my last outings. In just two days I am scheduled to fly from Buenos Aires to Johannesburg, South Africa, a ticket I reserved three months ago. My thought was that having planned flights would propel me forward. Instead, it paints my final days in the city with regret. Such a huge part of me wants to stay.

The stadium, La Bombonera, is located in La Boca, a working-class barrio with a colorful history. La Boca ("the mouth" in English) is located at the mouth of the Riachuelo river, which forms the southern border of Buenos Aires. The river is also the reason the neighborhood was formed—La Boca was settled by workers from the shipyards that dot the banks. The houses are crafted from shipping materials, like grainy, cast-off planks and corrugated metal, and painted with leftover supplies, so each facade is a different color, creating a wild patchwork display.

The neighborhood is rough, which is why we are under the watchful eye of a guide. She is there to sweep us past the police barricades and through a funnel of people into the stadium. We are told repeatedly that foreigners should not be alone in this neighborhood after dark—under no circumstances are we to come here by ourselves.

The bus drops us off on El Caminito, a cobblestoned street full of souvenir shops and art displays, like an open-air museum. Our escort gives us strict instructions to stick to the lit and well-traveled Caminito while we find food and restrooms, then to meet back at the bus in a half hour.

The buildings along the walkway are painted primary colors, so garish that they are beautiful. The colors are stacked like a child's blocks, one against the next. A blue wall leans into a yellow building, while red shutters sag along a green windowsill. Life-sized mannequins lean from the balconies, depicting the seedy history of this neighborhood in a jovial manner. Laughing prostitute mannequins are fondled by leering sailor dolls. Mafia mannequins look on.

On the corner, a real couple dances the tango. At the end of each song, the woman poses dramatically while her partner passes a black fedora and asks for tips. Painters display their art on chain-link fences; the work is textured and bright, matching the buildings that form a real-life backdrop. They look more like postcards than paintings.

Each restaurant has a patio, and the scent of food is overwhelming. Waiters carry sizzling steaks as round as a cocktail waitress's tray. Volcanoes of pasta erupt with oil and marinara sauce. The pizzas are tall, piled with shredded cheese and grilled vegetables. My stomach growls, and Jeff's stomach responds with a similar noise.

We can't resist the call of the restaurants—especially not when waiters tug on our arms, shove menus in our faces, promise us the most wonderful food in all of Argentina.

We sit at a table topped with a red-and-white tablecloth and are given bottled beers and a basket of fresh-baked bread. I end up with a platter of fresh ravioli, and the pasta is toothy enough to hold the cheese inside but soft enough to melt with each bite. It is slathered in a sage-and-butter sauce, salty and slippery and fatty. Jeff doesn't speak as he lingers over his own meal, a plate of gnocchi. Red sauce clings to the grooves of each potato dumpling, then to the stubble of his strong jaw.

Between the beers and the carbs, we lose track of time. By the time we pay for our meals and make it back to the spot where we were dropped off, the bus is gone.

"Shit," Jeff says. "What do we do now?"

We decide to find the street where La Bombonera is located—our tour group will have to pass by eventually. We can reconnect with them there, collect our tickets, and still have an escort to our seats.

Except, we realize after we find La Bombonera, our group might have already passed by. Dusk is quickly disappearing, shifting firmly into night, and I can't help but think that this might be a bad place to be waiting on a street corner in the dark.

Passersby walk in clusters, everybody wearing blue and gold clothes, scarves, and hats from head to toe. One chucks an empty can at me with impeccable aim, hitting me square in the chest. That's when I realize I am inadvertently wearing black and red, the colors of the rival team playing in tonight's game.

Instead of the street corner, Jeff and I retreat to the steps of a nearby bank. Even though it's closed, I figure banks have security cameras, and I feel slightly safer under a watchful electronic gaze.

"I don't feel so good about this," I say.

Jeff turns to me and hisses through clenched teeth. "Don't . . . speak . . . English," he says. "Not now."

So I am silent, and the time passes slowly. The chill of the concrete steps tears right through the denim of my rhinestoned jeans. I pull my black jacket tighter around my chest, try to cover the red shirt underneath. The sky is now navy, and street lamps flicker on. In my peripheral vision, I see my reflection in a long glass door that leads to the bank's ATM. I eye myself as if I'm a stranger, and I try to assess if I could pass for Argentinian. I wonder if I look like I belong. I see shadows in my face, but there's light there too.

Jeff is reflected in the glass next to me. He is tall, but so am I, and I wonder how many people we could take in a fight if it came to that.

The pasta sits heavy in my stomach. I am no longer hungry, just full of regret. I wish I had never seen the adorable table, the convincing waiter, the dumb ravioli that got us into this mess. Fireworks sizzle upward from the stadium and shoot into sparkles in the night sky. I hear the crowd chant and sing. The game is about to begin.

I almost don't believe my eyes when our tour escort crosses the street, the rest of our group in tow.

"It's them!" I say.

"Shhhh," Jeff warns.

"No, look." I'm so excited, I can't contain my volume. I leap to my feet. "It's them! Our group is here."

We run to catch up with them, and our escort is visibly relieved. And angry.

Mostly angry. She reluctantly hands over our tickets for the game.

"Stay by my side the rest of the night, both of you," she says, pointing her finger and waving it in the air as if it were a weapon. "Or else."

At the stadium, the stairs are sodden with liquid, and the concrete hallways smell of stale beer and urine. Our guide ushers us to our bleacher seats, which are tucked underneath an overhang filled with rowdy Boca Junior supporters.

"Stay underneath here," the tour guide says; then she points to the shouting, cheering, singing men above. "The fans like to pee on the tourists. Though you two," she points at Jeff and me. "I should let you get pissed on."

The football game is secondary to the action from the crowd. In front of me, a slurring man climbs rafters and, with a wobbly grip, hoists a Boca Junior banner in the air. The crowd cheers, even when he nearly stumbles and falls. Everybody seems to know the same songs, which are repeated throughout the match, and every chant booms like thunder beneath our seats. The effect is celebratory and colorful, and the festivities leave me unbelievably exhilarated. I don't even care who wins. I try to sing along, but I only catch every fourth word.

"I can't believe you're going to be in Africa, like, the day after tomorrow," Jeff says.

I suck in my breath. Even my lungs want to pause this moment and prolong my stay.

"I don't want to think about it," I say. "I mean, I'm excited to see South Africa, but I had no idea leaving this place would be so hard."

At that, the man and woman sitting in front of us turn and introduce themselves. Erin and Pete. They are a married couple from America.

"We're headed to South Africa in a few days too—" Erin says.

Pete finishes her sentence, "And we're looking for someone to travel with us."

I like them immediately. Pete is a teacher, with rumpled red hair and a nose dotted with freckles. Erin a lobbyist and lawyer, has a sleek brown bob and a friendly face, and she has been working for the same kind of liberal causes I support. We share the home state of Ohio. Erin is also a vegetarian, and Pete is fueled by coffee, just like me.

Navigating South Africa with a couple of nice Ohioans might not be the worst idea. Erin, Pete, and I agree to meet the next day to discuss our traveling styles, see if we might make a good backpacking fit.

Finally, the match is over—a Boca Junior win—and masses of people swarm the pitch. Flares send scarlet smoke into the sky, the color of autumn leaves. The guide tells us to wait under the overhang until security can assist us. Fights break out in the stairwells. Men pee all over their feet and all over each other; there's piss everywhere. It's a glorious, slovenly, drunken scene. When the tour guide says it is time to go, I am reluctant to leave.

This place is cluttered with litter. The crowd is noisy. I have no roots here. There are no ancestral springs in this land for me. Still I feel like my notion of home has already changed and stretched to include this part of the world, this city, this stadium, this night. Maybe I don't need to stay here, but I will carry this place with me as I move on.

One Straw Can Be Broken,
but Together They Are Strong

—⟨≋⟩—

I'm in a rented Nissan, headed to the Wild Coast of South Africa. My friends from the Argentinian football game are in the front—Erin is driving, and Pete is in the passenger seat. I'm in the backseat with Barbara, who wanted to travel with us for the next month.

The driving is slow. The road is rocky, caramel-colored dirt, slicing through mossy green hills. There are potholes on top of potholes, and Erin navigates the car carefully, but every once in a while, a tire still sinks into the road with a jarring thunk.

Every hillside is dotted with pastel-colored huts, round with pointy, thatched roofs, like something that would house a village full of charming gnomes. Animals graze in the pasture. Occasionally we pass a group of children playing in the nearby fields, and they run after our car, dancing in the dust kicked up by the tires. Their smiles are so wide, it makes me smile alongside them.

Suddenly Erin hits the brakes and we screech to a halt, barely missing a thin and energetic goat that has run into the road.

"Whew," I say. "That was a close one."

Erin begins to drive again, but within seconds, she slams on the brakes once more. This time, the car stops just before we run over a fat log. It's as wide as a stump and is attached to about ten feet of rope that encircles the tiny goat's neck. He is trotting along the road, dragging the log behind him.

I love that spunky goat—the little guy who so desperately wants to run free, he has yanked out the log that was supposed to restrain him. I love the fierce beauty of the scenery, the wild blue ocean that breaks just beyond the hills. I am the annoying tourist in the backseat, singing a 1980s Toto classic at the top of my lungs.

I am joyful to be here. I am grateful for this country, this continent. I lean my head against the seat and relax into this big love that began my first full day in South Africa and has only increased since.

That was the day I visited the Cradle of Humankind, a UNESCO World Heritage Site, about fifty kilometers northwest of Johannesburg. The area has produced some of the oldest pre-human remnants ever found, including the 2.3-million-year-old Mrs. Ples fossil, which was excavated from a nearby cave in 1947. She is that link between primate and *Homo sapiens*, believed to be a distant relative to all humankind.

There are many fossils similar to Mrs. Ples, all packaged in tidy boxes with thick glass, where visitors can look at them from every angle. Mrs. Ples herself isn't on display, but there are photos, drawings, and reconstructions of her skull. The entire effect is something cartoonish, her forehead slightly flattened, with a jutting bone beneath her nose, the way a chimpanzee's face presses out. Her eye sockets are perfectly oval, as if widened with surprise.

Somewhere along the way, Mrs. Ples became a mother to someone who became a mother to someone who became a mother. Then eventually, after many thousands of years, came my grandmother, and then my mother, and then me. A scientist would probably say it isn't that simple—but then again, it is. One woman begets another. Those of us who exist now carry the generations that came before us. I can almost feel this thread unspooling.

That idea alone makes me want to sing out and embrace the people around me. It helps chase away the isolation, the outsider-ness that I've felt elsewhere. If I am engaged with something bigger than I ever knew before, linked to a family so sprawling I don't know how to map it, I am part of a larger whole. I have many mothers.

It was late afternoon when I left the Cradle of Humankind museum. The vast savannah that surrounds the site glowed gold, nearly the same gold as my mother's hair. The dirt there is a strong red-brown, as if rich with the bones and blood of ancients. The trees are wispy and wide, their branches stretched open like patio umbrellas. I saw a thin snake in the long grass.

The air was warm and dry, and it reminded me of the desert I call home. I'd finally shed the fleece jacket I'd worn for three months straight in South America.

When I called my dad that night, I was just about to hang up when he said, "Wait!"

"Yes?"

"Africa," he said. "Is it pretty?"

The question brought tears to my eyes. South Africa is gorgeous, but it is also a feeling. One that I had no words for yet.

This was also the first time my dad had shown genuine interest in my trip. In three months, he'd never asked me a question about the place I was currently in. My mom must have been doing better, I assumed, for him to wonder about something else.

"Yes," I said, and I was grateful he'd asked. "It's very pretty."

ERIN, PETE, BARBARA, AND I SHARE A HUT ON THE WILD Coast at an eco-lodge called Bulungula, located in one of the most remote villages in South Africa, Nqileni.

Bulungula has minimal electricity, and there is no cell phone service or internet. There are showers, but they remain hot for approximately five minutes—about as long as the small paraffin furnace at the base of the shower remains lit. Bread is baked the traditional way, inside a dirt pit.

A coastal forest sprawls all the way to the sand of the estuary and kisses the edge. The water is a heart-stopping blue, true and bright and clear. At night, the sky is generously sprinkled with stars I've never seen before.

On our first full morning, an acrid scent hits my nose and at first I think there must be a landfill nearby. But when I walk the beach, a man from the nearby Xhosa village shows me the source of the odor.

"Dead whale," he says with a shrug, as if it happens all the time.

I nod and shrug in return, as if I should have known better.

The massive beast no longer looks like a whale. It is more like a smudge on the shore, its skin melting into the sand. The smell is briny and musky, fish and rot, dirty sex and earth. It is tinged with the sweetness of decay and the sourness of time. And despite my attempts to hold myself together, the odor makes me gag.

The mammal washed ashore about three weeks prior to my arrival, but I didn't smell it right off. This morning the wind shifted, carrying the smell right up to the door of my hut.

The nearby villagers have already extracted much of the carcass, sawing off layers of fat, meat, organs. The remnants remain on the surf, discarded blubber and bone, bleached by the sun, washed by the waves. The beast is slowly returning to the sea, piece by piece.

I take photos, crouching close enough to the whale that it looks like rock strata through my lens—layers of blue, white, and brown folded onto one another. The villager on the beach watches me and erupts into laughter.

"I can show you more dead animals," he says with a smile.

It's funny, but it's yet another reminder that I'm just a voyeur here. To me, this whale is a snapshot for a photo album. For another, the whale carcass is survival.

This use of the whale flesh makes me think about my mom's family in Europe during World War II, scavenging potatoes from already-picked-over fields, sucking the juice from bones that had already been boiled. They ate whatever they could, anything to cobble together an existence. I wonder what my mom would have done if some stranger had snapped photos of the experience.

The thought makes me uncomfortable, and for the first time on this trip,

I put my camera away. I simply stand on the beach with the man, and I watch the water crash over the whale's broken and exposed body, every wave taking away another piece.

THERE ARE MANY ACTIVITIES TO DO IN THE VILLAGE, AND I choose to spend a day with Abalene, a woman from Nqileni. She brings me to the hut where she and her sister live.

Abalene pours water into a bowl of dry clay and stirs it gently with her fingers. Then she spreads it on my face, smoothing the brown mud over my cheeks, forehead, nose, and chin. It's been a while since I've had someone else's hands on me. It feels both intimate and strange, like the first tentative touch of a new lover. I close my eyes and take it in. The longer she strokes my face, the more maternal it feels.

A memory surfaces of an incident that took place around 2005, about a year before my mom entered the nursing home. My dad was away for a work trip, so I was Mom's caregiver for the weekend. I had to give her a bath, because she could no longer take showers on her own. There was the fear that she could slip and fall, of course, but more importantly, on a couple of occasions my mom had tried to bring a plugged-in hair dryer into the running shower. "My hair was getting wet," she explained.

At this point, Mom was still in one of the earlier stages of the disease— too far gone to know my name but cognizant enough to know I was someone trying to help. She was also stubborn enough to fight.

It's difficult enough to give your own mother a bath—it's a vulnerable act for everyone involved—but it's even harder when she doesn't want to do it. She thrashed, spilling bathwater on the floor, and she cried, spilling tears everywhere. I sat on the tile with my back against the door until she calmed enough to stay in the tub.

I bribed her with lovely, lilac-scented soap, then whispered, "Shhh," as I wiped down her skin with a washcloth. Without her clothes, she looked very small. I smoothed her face with my fingers, cupped her chin in my hand. She was no longer crying, but her body hiccuped with silent sobs.

Abalene's sister picks up another bowl—this one smaller than the first—and holds a matchstick between her thumb and index finger. She dips the end of the matchstick in reddish clay, drawing a line of dots around my forehead, then another line across my cheekbones and the bridge of my nose. On each cheek she makes small, swishy lines, fashioning simple daisies. She is the artist, and I am her canvas.

The clay face paint is part decorative, like local cosmetics, but it's also practical. We're going to be spending most of the day in the sun. The clay will act as a natural sunblock for my fair skin.

Abalene also grabs a red scarf and wraps it around my hair, tugging the curls into the fabric, then drawing both ends of the scarf into a knot, which she situates near the top of my head.

I hold my camera in front of my face and shoot a self-portrait, then examine the image. I don't recognize the face staring back at me. The first layer of clay has dried mint green, while the design is a ruddy red. I look beautiful but different, as if the Wild Coast has ripped away my surface and left me with something new.

Abalene smiles. With her approval, we head outside.

She teaches me to scavenge from the nearby forest, gathering firm sticks for firewood. This will be our kindling later when we prepare lunch. We secure the bundles with strips of fabric. Abalene places a bundle on top of my head, and I lean and sway from the sudden weight and strange pressure.

"Stand up tall," she says. "Hold head high."

I feel a knot of gnarled wood knuckling into my head, and I also feel the place where wood splinters catch on my red head scarf. All the sticks are long and hard, and when I walk, they threaten to topple. As I become more sure-footed, however, the branches also grow more confident. The wood perches as if it were meant to be there, like the branches were sprouting from my head.

I slowly, slowly make my way back up the hill and into Abalene's hut. I don't drop the wood, not even a single stick. She smiles and claps.

"Now let us try a bucket of water on your head," she says.

The bucket ends up at my feet, my right shoulder baptized. A group of village children hoot, and I can't help but giggle with them. Water drips down my side; clay runs along the side of my face. Abalene and I wipe tears from our eyes, we are laughing so hard.

"This is why you have the small bucket," she says.

ABALENE'S HOME BECOMES MY OWN FOR THE DAY. I KNEEL on the compacted dirt floor, where I use a flat stone to grind corn into course pieces, like dry grits. Abalene has already cooked a pot of beans, which she sets aside while she boils water. We talk and she cooks the cornmeal until it becomes a thick porridge called *ugali*.

"You cook?" Abalene says, and I nod.

"Yes, but never ugali."

"Then what do you eat?" she asks, incredulously.

The ugali is stiffer than day-old mashed potatoes. We roll it into balls with our fingers, then use the balls to sop up the bean stew. Until now, Abalene's son, a child about four years old, has been playing in a neighbor's hut. Now he sits close to me on the floor, his legs slung over mine.

While we eat, Abalene tells me about her family. Her husband works in the mineral mines near Johannesburg, several hours away. Like most of the men in this village, he leaves for months at a time. This leaves the women to run the town. They raise and educate the children. They care for each other's farms. They tend to the sick and the elderly together. When one person's cow wanders from the field, every woman sets off to search for it.

There's an old saying in South Africa that a single straw from a broom can be broken, but together they are strong. That concept is known as *ubuntu*, the philosophy that we are all part of an interconnected web, rooted in acts of kindness and generosity. It means the way we treat others is more important than our individual accomplishments. Essentially, you can't be human all by yourself.

I think about ubuntu a lot in this village, because I see it in action. Abalene breaks off a piece of bread to share with her young son. He toddles to the door, where he has three friends waiting. There he tears the bread and gives a piece to each of his friends.

Abalene pokes her head out the door and calls to a handful of women washing clothes in buckets outside a nearby hut. They saunter over and share some of the bean stew and ugali. As they leave, Abalene hands them a small stack of her laundry, which they will wash with their own.

We clean the dishes by hand, and I stack the bowls on a small table. That's when I notice a framed photo on the wall, a black-and-white image of a finely dressed woman, head held high like royalty, eyes small and firm. I look to Abalene, and she answers before I ever ask the question.

"Mother," she says.

I pull my iPhone from my bag. It doesn't receive any service out here, but I can still access the photo library. I scroll through the photos, showing Abalene my best friend, my husband, my brother, my sister.

I stop when I get to a blonde woman, her head raised high just like Abalene's mother, curls framing her face like a halo. She is sitting on a park bench in Europe, slim legs crossed at the knees, the hem of her checkered dress flared out around her calves. Her lips are slightly pouty, frozen mid-word.

This woman looks past the camera, far beyond the photographer. Sometimes I wonder what she is thinking in that long-distance gaze, if she can somehow see beyond that moment. Imaginary loves, future sorrows, a home across the ocean.

"Mother?" Abalene says.

I nod.

"Beautiful," Abalene says. "She looks like you."

IN THE LATE AFTERNOON, THE SUN GROWS HEAVY AND VI-olet. Abalene walks me over to the local shebeen. It is a small bar situated inside a sea-green hut, three hills over from Abalene's home.

Though shebeens are where people drink alcohol, they also serve as community spaces—meeting places where people share conversation and dance. During the apartheid era, activists gathered in shebeens to share news and make plans with the community.

Abalene does not enter. She says she has a lot of things to do this evening.

Instead, she hugs me and wishes me well. This is where we will part ways for the night.

Inside, the walls are plain. The hut feels much bigger than Abalene's home even though it is filled with people. Most everyone sits on the floor, legs stuck out in front of them, feet bare and brown. The patrons are divided into two groups, just like a junior high school dance—men on one side of the room, women on the other.

It takes a few minutes before I notice that the men are of varying ages, from teenagers to withered old men. However, there are no young women in the shebeen, only older ladies. This, I will later learn, is because many women of childbearing age refrain from alcohol, in case they might be pregnant.

One woman hikes up her skirt and dances wildly in the middle of the room. Her face is crackly and dry, the texture of course sandpaper, with firm lines like parentheses on each side of her mouth. She spins like a top, never losing balance, but never remaining fully upright either. Then she stops and abruptly focuses her yellowed eyes on my face, as if she has just noticed me for the first time. She motions to me, and her friend slings a paint can full of *umqombothi*, sorghum beer, my way.

I lift the can but pause before I take a sip. The smell is overpowering, like fermented fruit and sour pork. I peer down into the can and examine the thick, brownish-pink liquid. The old dancing lady cackles. Her friends join in, laughing until the room is wheezy. Then the men encourage me to drink with their clapping and hollering.

I tip the can toward my face. The frothy liquid is viscous and it moves slowly, the same way diner ketchup crawls slowly through a glass bottle. Just when I think I'll never get a taste, the beer abruptly rushes at me at once, staining my lips, dribbling down my chin, even smearing my cheeks. Only a little umqombothi makes it into my mouth, just barely enough to swallow, and I am thankful for that. It is a bitter porridge and tastes of vomit, acidic and sweet. The shebeen erupts into cheers as I wipe the remnants of the drink from my face. I receive hugs and slaps on the back, and I'm amazed that I can be congratulated for simply accepting something to drink. My stomach gurgles with discomfort.

There are many types of drinking, and I've tried most of them over the years. There's the kind of drinking that's done to forget pain and heartbreak. There's the kind of drinking that's done out of boredom, a way to live through one hour and then the next. There's drinking to be social and drinking to be snobby and drinking to be joyfully drunk and drinking to wrestle with an inner beast.

But this kind—slugging back umqombothi in a shebeen—is a particular type of drinking I have never experienced before. It is a cultural drink that tastes bitter and terrible and staggeringly complex, a welcome into a community at the edge of an unknown country. It's warmth. Maybe that's why I feel flushed.

I leave the shebeen close to dark, when the silver moon is swollen over the estuary, lighting the bloated carcass of the whale. The beer in my stomach is heavy and clanging. The evening has been a contract, an understanding, a shared experience between strangers.

I haven't spent much time here, but I already feel like one among many. Is this what my mother longed to feel? Is this why she wanted to travel? Her childhood was spent displaced by war, moving from East Prussia to what eventually became West Germany. Her life with my father was spent hop-scotching around the United States, moving from military base to military base. Is this feeling what inspired her wanderlust? Did she just want to find a space to belong?

Animals

———⊗⊗⊗———

AFTER NEARLY A MONTH IN SOUTH AFRICA, I HAVE HIKED
up Table Mountain, sampled the hottest curries in Durban, found sisterhood
in the huts of the Wild Coast, and stood on the farthest tip of Africa while
the sturdy winds whipped my hair across my face. Now I'm ready for a safari.
This is another one of the things my mom wanted to do in her life.

After leaving the Wild Coast, Erin, Pete, Barbara, and I head to Kruger
National Park for five days of camping, after which we will drive to Johannesburg together and part ways.

Kruger is remarkable, a sprawling park larger than Israel, making it one
of the largest game reserves in all of Africa. It's impossible to navigate in just
a few days, so we have reserved campsites at three different locations in the
park.

We have two tents. Erin and Pete share one; Barbara and I take the
other. The tents are shaped like Frisbees. Unzip one side, toss the whole
thing on the ground, and the tent pops up like magic. They are small and

leaky—Barbara and I have lined ours with duct tape—and they barely shield us from the icy nighttime wind. But since all of us are on tight budgets, this is where we sleep most nights, at cheap campsites throughout South Africa.

The roads in the park are high quality, so our days are spent in the rented Nissan, looping through Kruger's fourteen different ecozones on self-drive safaris. We see the Big Five of game animals—lion, African elephant, Cape buffalo, leopard, and rhinoceros—several times over, in addition to other wildlife.

On a densely wooded roadside, I observe the slit mouth of a cheetah as it dozes beneath a tree. Erin stops the car for a hippopotamus, which is almost as wide as the road. We see crocodiles and warthogs, leaping herds of kudu and zeals of zebras, a wake of vultures feasting on a giraffe carcass.

At night, I am the cook for our group, making one-pot meals in the campsite kitchens. Packages of dried ramen noodles mixed with canned vegetables. Boiled pasta with a tin of spaghetti sauce. Rice and beans. This is the food I ate in college, when I couldn't afford anything fresh.

Every morning, Pete and I stir crystals of instant coffee into hot water and curl our frigid fingers around the warm mugs. His is a takeout cup, saved from a fast-food joint where we stopped earlier in the month. Mine is a travel mug from Addo Elephant Park that has held everything from hot coffee to cold beer.

Sometimes I hold the coffee and close my eyes, thinking of all the lazy mornings I spent at home with Jason, sprawled out in bed, reading the Sunday paper, and drinking black coffee. When I get too sad, I push through those memories, open my eyes, and focus on the wildlife that surrounds me instead.

Some of the other campers tease my friends and me. Other groups are well equipped with elaborate tents, rented RVs, lounge chairs, inflatable mattresses, coolers full of beer, gas grills, tiny refrigerators that plug into the cigarette lighter of a Land Cruiser.

But I like the way I'm experiencing this country. My blood tolerates coldness better, and my skin is slightly harder. I have not looked in a mirror for weeks. Every night I feel the dirt of Africa beneath my back. The ground is so firm, so complete, sometimes I think it's cradling me.

TWO DAYS LATER, WE HAVE MADE IT HALFWAY THROUGH the park.

I sit in a wildlife blind, tiger stripes of light across my face. Surrounding me are animals I've only read about before. A group of elephants coat themselves in mud by a water hole. They fling dirt at each other playfully, stir the earth with their trunks.

My ears are filled with birdsong, and I smell sweet grass, sun-warmed leaves, the musk of large animals. The land is expansive, and I've never seen anything so great or so wide before. There is a rain cloud in the distance, but I know it might never reach me here.

All the unkempt feelings I had in South America, all the times I felt aimless or that I didn't belong—I don't have those emotions here. This country is giving me something I didn't know how to ask for. Though I'm here with three others, it's rare to be in a place where animals outnumber people, and I like being in this minority. This specific type of isolation is seductive and comforting.

I watch herds of animals come and go to the water hole, and I think about home. It's impossible to reach my family from the bushveld, with no internet service for many miles. But even if I could call them right now, what would I say?

The farther I travel, the more distance I feel from my family. My dad holds his cell phone so close to my mom's ear that I hear the thud of the phone making contact with her hearing aid. I tell her where I am. I tell her what I'm seeing, the things I'm doing, how I'm feeling. I tell her that I miss her. But the one-sidedness of the conversation makes me ache.

Even connected, there is disconnect. While I used to receive some response—sometimes a mumble, more often a groan—now she doesn't answer at all. I strain for something between the hum of the phone line and the scritch of her hearing aid. She gives me no words, only her silence. She's the one disappearing, but it's as though the disease has erased me.

Does she remember the yellow rocking chair from our living room, the place where she soothed my worries and held me until my nightmares disappeared? Does she know we had a fight when she found a pack of cigarettes in my purse? Does she hold any memories of us at all? My clarinet recitals, our shopping trips, the nights we stayed up late talking about everything and nothing?

I wish I knew if I were situated at all within the folds of her brain. Does she ever have visions of a frizzy-haired little girl, round-bellied and pink from the sun, and wonder why she's there? Does she see ghosts of me, the same way my mind conjures visions of her, of how things used to be? Do I shadow dance across the walls of her mind?

Sometimes I have trouble remembering her before the disease. That's one of the most brutal things about Alzheimer's: it didn't just take my mom; it has done a "find and replace" on my own recollections. The bulk of my memories of Mom are in the context of illness: confused in our house, confused at the nursing home, the times she forgot where she was going, the times she got violent and angry because she didn't know who we were or why we were in her room.

If I try hard to summon her and dive deep in my memories, I emerge with senses instead of scenes: the sound of her crooning along with Elvis in the car, the scalp-tickling sensation of her playing with my hair, the scent of her citrusy 4711 cologne. These are the memories that have been stored in the body, the animal-like relationship between a mother and daughter. It takes real work for me to conjure anything more precise. The longer she is sick, the more she slips away.

Inventor Thomas Edison believed that memory was a factory, and there were tiny workers who stashed information away into the Broca's area, part of the frontal-lobe region of the brain. When a person had trouble recalling something, it simply meant the worker responsible for that particular memory was on break and couldn't retrieve it. Conversely, to remember something is to get in touch with the shift that was on duty at the time the memory was recorded. I know Edison's theory isn't true, but I think about it a lot. Sometimes I imagine my factory workers are out to lunch or tipsy. My mom's factory, though, has been gutted.

From the wildlife blind, I watch an adult giraffe stretch for leaves on a tree. Suddenly a baby giraffe trots out from behind it and runs to his mother. He nudges beneath her knobby legs and stands in her shadow.

Although baby giraffes hit the ground feetfirst and walk almost immediately, I know mama giraffes care for their young as long as necessary— sometimes as long as sixteen months—to teach them survival skills. The mature males leave the group they were born into and can spend their entire lives alone. But the females tend to stay together in small groups. They bond.

Now the top of the young one's head grazes the pale, fine fur of his mother's belly. Together the giraffes almost seem to be an eight-legged figure, two shapes combined into one. I yearn for that. I am just an animal, after all. I want to run to my mom, seek the protection of her body. But I am motherless now, even while she still breathes.

Does the fact that my mother can no longer care for me mean that I'm equipped to navigate this world on my own? If that's the law of nature, why does it feel so unnatural?

OUR FINAL NIGHT IN KRUGER, THE WIND HAS FANGS.
We pitch our tents under the shelter of a few trees, near a chain-link fence with a sign that warns against feeding the hyenas.

The spotted animals patrol the length of the fence anyway. Though they are still wild, these hyenas have grown accustomed to humans here and seem unafraid.

Our neighbors are boisterous and drunk Afrikaners. They set up a pop-up tent on top of a hulking Land Rover. They drag patio furniture onto the grass, pull out a grill, light the charcoal. They cook *boerewors* sausage coils and thick steaks, foil-wrapped potatoes and a pot of soupy beans, then toss their meat scraps over the fence. The hyenas fight for the gristle and skin.

My friends and I want to celebrate Halloween, even though the holiday isn't known here.

I learned this earlier in the day, when we checked into the campsite. I asked the ranger if there were any Halloween activities for the park's international guests. He said he has never heard of Halloween before.

"It's a holiday," I said. "In America, we celebrate it by dressing up in costumes, knocking on neighbors' doors, and asking for candy."

"And they give it to you?"

"Yes. Because if they don't, you can play a mean trick on them."

"I don't understand," he said. "Why would you do that?"

I hadn't thought about it before, and I didn't know how to respond. After a long pause I explained, "Because Halloween is all about being scary. A lot of people dress up like vampires, witches, zombies, mummies—anything dead. And then they frighten other people."

"Dead things?"

My explanation wasn't adequate, and he didn't get it. We dropped the Halloween talk and focused on the registration process instead. When that was finished, I turned to walk away. The ranger yelled cheerfully after me, "Have a nice Halloween! I hope you drown in a swimming pool tonight!"

For our own festivities, Pete and I decide to be our Afrikaner neighbors, quietly and out of earshot. We hike our pants up to our ribs, hoist our beers in the air, and try on South African accents, bragging about our fat boerewors and how we're going to cook it on the *braai*. Then Barbara pretends to be a lion and chases us around our tents.

"Happy Halloween!" Pete hands me a piece of candy from our food supplies.

It's hard to believe this is one of our final nights together. Barbara is headed to Madagascar, where she'll be working on a lemur census. Erin and Pete are on a fast track through East Africa, zipping through Uganda and Rwanda before heading to Egypt. And I'm also going to Uganda, but I am in for a longer stay—I'm still in the process of making plans, but I'll likely volunteer on a farm in exchange for a place to sleep.

After dinner, we are too cold to stay outside, even though we want to prolong our time together. We crawl into our tents, and the drunk neighbors wander into our campsite and jeer. "It's too cold for your tents!" they yell, as if we have a choice of accommodations for the night. "You need a strong one like ours."

The wind howls through the duct-taped seams of the tent, and my summer sleeping bag does little to keep me warm. I pull on a hat and some gloves. The frame of our tent buckles and sways with every gust.

"I feel like the wind is talking to us," Barbara says. It does almost sound like whistles and chirps. I strain to listen to what it's saying but I can't make out the words. Eventually I fall into the kind of unsettled sleep that feels like slipping on cobblestones; every time I'm about to tumble, I wake with a jolt.

I don't know what time it is when I hear the crack. It shatters the blackness of night. Then a boom. A crash. I have no idea what's happening. Uncertainty grips me.

I hear Barbara's breath quicken. We are both still with fear. My eyes water as they always do when my body is tight with terror, and I wipe the tears away.

"Should we go outside?" Barbara says.

"I don't know," I say. The wind moans; then it's joined by animal chatter. From my tent, I see a flashlight. The light is yellow, but the canvas walls filter it into a delicate green. I hear another tent unzip.

A moment later, our tent shakes.

"Guys," Pete says. "Come out and see."

I strap my headlamp around my forehead and flick on the light before I crawl out of the tent. Outside, everything looks different than it did earlier, and I flounder to make sense of the scene.

The campground looks like a dense jungle. Leaves rattle. The sky is streaked with the first bluish lines of morning light, and wind rushes across my face. There are fallen branches everywhere. Where the neighbors' grill and patio furniture used to be, there is now a tree.

On closer inspection with our flashlight beams, my friends and I see that an entire tree didn't fall against the Land Rover. However, a sizable portion of it did, as though the wind cracked the tree right in half.

The neighbors carefully step out of their pop-up tent on the car roof and climb down the ladder attached to the vehicle's side, the metal now tangled with branches. The Afrikaners are dazed, but safe. We help them find a place to sit, away from the mess of sticks and leaves. Erin brings them water.

The fallen tree only narrowly missed crashing through their tent. After it hit the roof, the thick limbs rolled off the vehicle and onto the patio furniture, shattering it all. The tree came close to crushing the chain-link fence—the one thing that separates us from the scavengers.

The animals are here now, summoned by the clatter and the light. The hyenas stand in a line, watching us beasts with unblinking, round eyes. I stare back, and I wonder if I am as strange to them as they are to me. The fence looks more delicate than it ever did before, almost like filigree. The line that separates us from wildness is so thin, it's almost not there at all.

Honor Your Tribe

———— ⌘ ————

IT'S LATE AFTERNOON IN KAMPALA, UGANDA, WHEN I CALL my dad's cell phone. It is 8 a.m. in Ohio, and my mom is being fed powdered eggs.

"I'm trying to decide where to go next," I tell my dad.

"That's nice," he says.

My laptop rests on top of my knees while I sit cross-legged on a hostel's red-painted porch, which opens out into a large plot of land. From my perch I see a pig almost as big as a loveseat, groups of cartwheeling monkeys, and lines of laundry strung up but sagging from the humidity.

"I want to do something that helps people," I say to my dad. "I found this farm ..."

"That sounds like a good idea," he says.

He is distracted, possibly resentful. The last time he showed interest in my travels was a month ago, when he asked if Africa was pretty.

My dad didn't encourage me to take this trip—he wanted me to stay at my job until I earned my retirement and a gold watch from the company. He is a man who doesn't believe in quests, quitting jobs, or movement without a safety net. He does believe in rules, structure, and a guaranteed paycheck. He also believes loyalty is still rewarded with gold watches. But once I made my decision, he accepted it, even though it meant slapping another layer of worry onto his life.

Some of the travelers camp here on the scraggly lawn, but I've been sleeping on a bunk bed in a sweaty room. A three-legged black-and-white kitten has befriended me and clambers into my bed every night. I think he knows I'm lonely.

My dad is obviously distracted with caring for my mom, so I sign off.

"Well, I'm probably headed to this place called Freddie's Farm. I'll call when I get there," I say. "Tell mom I love her, okay?"

I found Freddie on the internet when I searched for nonprofits in East Africa that need volunteers—his farm was described as a social-development project, ensuring food security for people in Eastern Uganda. Though his organization had good reviews from former workers, it was the photos of people laughing in rice fields that really attracted me.

Freddie asks for just twenty-five dollars a week to pay for lodging, which is less expensive than staying in a guesthouse. Not only will I be saving money, I'm looking forward to camaraderie and to feeling like part of a community again. While it was terrific to zip through South Africa in just one month, now I want to slow down, make friends, and become acquainted with one place for longer than a few days.

Freddie and I trade several emails before I arrive. I tell him I've never worked a field before, and Freddie reassures me. You don't need to be the best farmer or the quickest one, he writes. You just need to be present.

"Anything you can do will help," he insists. "We just need you."

He says if I don't like the field work, I can always teach children a new, sustainable method of planting banana trees.

"I don't know how to plant banana trees," I clarify.

"You will learn," he responds. "Please come."

I feel necessary in a way I haven't for months, which is enough to get me on the next bus from the capital city to rural Mbale, located on the eastern side of the country, near the border of Kenya. This is my first real excursion in Africa alone, and already I'm taking a bus across the country to meet a stranger on the other end. I'm pretty sure I know what awaits me in Mbale, but I can't be certain.

A man sits next to me on the bus, and he verbalizes some of my lingering doubts. "Why are you going to Mbale? There's nothing there. Who are you staying with? Do you even know what you're doing?"

My response sounds like an entry in *Lonely Planet*—and that's because everything I know about Mbale came from a guidebook.

"Well, it's the agricultural hub of Uganda, so I hear the markets are big and nice," I say. "It's a thriving provincial city with a superb setting at the bottom of Mount Elgon. And the terrain is beautiful. There are waterfalls and coffee plantations…"

"Sure?" the man says. It's a Ugandan vocal tick, administered in the same tone that an incredulous Californian might say, "Seriously?"

The man says that if it weren't for his family, he would never visit Mbale again. I try to change the subject.

"What's the best restaurant in town?" I ask.

"There is food."

"No. The best," I say. "What restaurant has the *best* meal?"

"The restaurants have food," he says. "There is no best."

Maybe we have a failure to communicate. Or maybe this man is telling me the truth. Maybe I'm in store for a bleak place. I rest my head on the scratched glass of the bus window and watch Kampala's smog and congestion slither away, replaced by the swaying grasses and red clay of the countryside.

The trees are tall enough to form a canopy over the road, their trunks hairy with vines. It reminds me of one particular gravel road that leads to my aunt's farm in southern Indiana, even though I'm sure the species of trees differ.

My husband once told me that the brain is always seeking patterns, because it doesn't like what it doesn't already know. That's why people see faces and animals and shapes in clouds—because our brains are trying to create something familiar out of the senseless and unknown. This is what I'm doing through the smeary bus window, imprinting a road I've traveled many times onto a foreign landscape.

It's beautiful enough that I should be at ease, but my stomach clenches anyway. What's going to happen to me in this place? I talk myself down by reminding myself of all the people I love back home—the reason why I'm taking this journey in the first place.

I don't think Uganda was ever on my mom's list, but her spirit is here. She wanted to live a more adventurous life and explore places she had never been before. And aren't I doing just that?

Hours later we reach the bus depot, a small stop on a dirt street. The structures vary in size, constructed of brick and bright paint. A few of them just look like skeletons, skinny boards and beams, the bones of a building. Motorcycles scream down the street, and cars kick up red dust. Vendors sell bottles of soda, and a lean man on the corner slices long stalks of sugarcane into bite-sized pieces to bag and sell. Children huddle at his feet, waiting for castoffs.

While I wait for my backpack to be unloaded from the undercarriage of the bus, my seatmate stands next to me, even though he isn't waiting for any luggage. He offers a final piece of unsolicited advice.

"You should know the bus leaves for Kampala many times a day," he says. "This afternoon, in fact."

"Thank you, but I don't think I'll be going so soon," I say. "I'm here for a purpose."

"Sure?"

I am not, but I nod anyway.

To get to Freddie's house, I take a short ride in a *matatu* minivan taxi, followed by a ride on a motorcycle taxi called a *boda-boda*, and then I walk a mile down a dirt road cluttered with goats and women balancing sacks of grain on their heads. His house is at the end of the road, a simple stone-and-brick ranch-style structure.

I knock, and Freddie comes to the screen door. He looks exactly like the photos online, tall and skinny, about thirty years old. His hair is closely cropped, and he wears crisp black pants and a long-sleeve shirt even though the weather is steamy.

He's so warm and welcoming, I don't hesitate to walk inside his house when he opens the door.

The living room is painted bright green. On one side of the room is a floral-pattered couch and a small TV, propped up on a plastic stool. On the other side of the room are rain barrels filled with rice.

Down the hallway, two bedrooms are lined with bunk beds and mosquito nets for volunteers. Freddie sleeps in the back of the house, a third bedroom. The kitchen is small and holds sacks of grain, a small, campfire-sized paraffin stove, and a dorm room–sized mini refrigerator. The bathroom has a toilet, but it doesn't flush, and there's a cold-water faucet for taking bucket showers.

I ask about the farm. Freddie says it's somewhere off-site. I guzzle purified water from my bottle while we talk, and I feel sweat beading on my upper back and rolling down my spine.

"We can go there another day," he says.

Only one other volunteer is staying with Freddie at the moment. Katie is a Canadian who has been living in Rwanda for six months, building websites for small businesses to fund travels throughout Africa. She says she's here for research—she's writing a guide to volunteer opportunities in East Africa.

I ask when I can start picking rice. It's so hot, and I'm already tired from the long day of travel, so I secretly hope Freddie won't say my volunteer work begins today.

"No, no rice," he says. "Harvest is done."

"No rice?"

"Next year," he says. "We'll have more."

"Oh. So I'll be teaching kids about planting banana trees then?" I say.

"The kids are on holiday," he says. "They have time away to help parents with the crops that have been harvested."

"No students?"

"No students," he confirms.

If there's no rice to harvest and no students to teach, why am I here? I told the man on the bus that I have a purpose, and now I guess that's a lie.

Freddie uses a paraffin stove on the floor to heat a pot of milk tea. He pours some into a chipped blue mug and hands it to me. It's too hot to drink, so I just hold it while I pace the floor.

"Relax," he says. "What else can you do?"

"I have no idea."

When it comes right down to it, what *can* I do? The skills of a journalist are about as useless in Mbale as a screen door on a submarine. I can't build a house or tend the sick. I can't help anyone with their crops or teach a new skill. All I can do is research stories and write articles for daily deadlines—which doesn't seem useful when I say it to Freddie in his living room.

"You are journalist?" he says. "Have you been on radio?"

I have. But only as a guest for local talk shows. I don't have any experience in radio production.

"Can you speak like a Southerner?" he says.

"Like, southern Ugandan?"

"No," he says. "Like Garth Brooks."

"Um," I pause. "I guess so."

When I pepper my speech with "y'all"s and a "bless yer heart," Freddie asks me to exaggerate my words and make the Southern twang more pronounced. When I sound like an approximation of Dolly Parton, Freddie declares it perfect.

It turns out that in addition to running an organic farm, Freddie is also a popular radio DJ and controls afternoon programming at the biggest FM station in this region. I didn't realize country music was so hot in Uganda, but Freddie quickly ticks off a list of performers: "Kenny Chesney, Shania Twain, Tim McGraw, Willie Nelson, Garth Brooks," he says. "We love them all. Especially the Garth Brooks."

The fact that many people in Mbale don't speak English is not a problem, Freddie says. "The people very much enjoy the soft sounds of Southern talking." And so he asks me to take on a different kind of volunteer task here—that of a country-western DJ at the radio station where he works.

The next day I receive a tour of the station, and Freddie's co-workers walk me through the job. I record promotional spots—"Y'all have been listening to STEP-FM, where country music matters"—and introduce "new" songs from Nashville, which are actually old songs from Nashville. We play The Oak Ridge Boys and Alabama, topped off with cuts from *Ultimate Clint Black*.

I don't know if anyone understands the words I am putting out into the air, but I guess it doesn't matter. I imagine my voice filling strangers' homes, and I like it. I picture the words as blue and silky, threading into someone else's ear, weaving us together. My mother is squelched and silenced by a disease, but my community grows with each word I send out over the airwaves.

The radio station also gives me the opportunity to use my journalism skills. As one of my first assignments, I interview a man who won a motorbike in a soda company's national contest. It sounds like a fluff story, something light that pads the real news. Then I meet the man.

He is young but unemployed and not by choice. When he does find work, it is poorly paid casual labor, never anything long-term. Now, with a motorbike, this man can start his own business by turning it into a boda-boda. Drivers are self-employed and usually make between seven and twenty dollars per day. This isn't just a simple win for him—it is the opportunity to change his life.

As a woman who has been spoiled by taxis, buses, cars, and traffic laws, bodas are terrifying. Nobody wears a helmet in Uganda, and a ten-minute ride through the city makes for many close calls as the boda pushes through tangles of traffic, tears over potholed dirt roads, and weaves through unruly farm animals.

When I arrived in Uganda, I was told that most people in the hospital are there as a result of boda-boda accidents, so I promised myself that I would never take a boda. No way. It was too unsafe, too unpredictable.

I will not take a boda.

Except I had to go to town to get a new electrical converter for my plugs. And no other vehicles went to that section of town.

Okay, just this one time. But definitely not again.

But bodas are faster, cheaper, and more convenient than matatus, the minivan taxis. Not to mention that they're a whole lot more comfortable. The matatus are licensed to carry fourteen people at a time, but they often squeeze in many more. Some of my rides have been uncomfortably hot and sticky, with twenty-six people and some fat goats.

Fine. I'll take bodas, but not at night.

And then one evening, there was no other way to get where I was going. *Bodas it is.*

Covering the story of this man's motorbike win gives me a new appreciation for the workers who drive through the congested city, out to the overgrown coffee fields, and back again, circling the entire region many times a day to support their families.

MBALE IS SO FAR FROM HOME, SOMETIMES I DON'T THINK of it at all. Concerns about my mother, questions about my future, and longing for my husband all seem to disappear into grassy fields and brick-colored streets. The city is walkable and friendly, and the days are filled with yolk-yellow light and cloudless skies. The people I meet are kind and inquisitive, curious how I ended up in Mbale.

I've seen one other white person in town, a man from Sweden, but everybody seems to think we know each other. I am stopped on the street by people who say, "I saw your brother! He went that way," and after a while I give up trying to explain that I don't know this man.

One afternoon, on my walk to the radio station, I take an alternate path, cutting between two houses instead of walking around the entire block.

A woman, squatting next to her house and washing a pan in a bucket, watches me until I am almost past; then she shouts, "Stop!"

I do, even though I am afraid I'm going to get in trouble for trespassing. "What is your name, woman?" she says, but not unkindly.

"Maggie."

She repeats my name slowly, letting it roll around on her tongue like warm gravy. "Maggie. Is that a shortcut for Margaret?"

I'm surprised she knows this, and I smile. "It is."

"What a coincidence," she says. Her face breaks into a grin too. "I could use a friend named Margaret."

The woman yells for her family, all of whom come outside and collect in a line by the side of the house. She introduces me as her new friend, and everybody reaches out a hand to shake mine.

I am invited inside for soupy beans and *posho*, cornmeal cooked until it is thick and stiff; it's like the ugali in South Africa, but with the addition of cassava flour. I can't stay long—I am expected to be back at the radio station within an hour—but I also don't want to be rude. It is so touching to be asked into someone's home, a generous invitation I can't refuse.

The woman's house looks nothing like my aunt's farmhouse in Indiana, but it smells just the same. Salt and broth and yeast and warm spices. The floor is cool, just compacted earth, and someone gives me a small mustard-yellow mat to sit on.

When the woman hands me a plate of food, I understand that I am supposed to eat the posho with my hands and use it to sop up the beans. With my left hand balancing the plate on my knees and my right hand sloppy with food, a lock of my hair falls into my face. A young girl, maybe ten years old, leans close to me. She brushes the hair from my forehead and tucks the curl behind my ear.

The tenderness of the gesture makes me want to cry. I could lie down here and fall asleep, happy and safe. I feel like a member of a family again.

It hits me for the first time that when my mom dies, I will be losing family in the way I've always known it. Though we will continue after she's gone, our family will only be the remains of something that once was. We will always yearn to be whole again.

Before I leave, the woman rubs my cheek and gives me a kiss on the forehead. What a coincidence, I think as I leave—I have been looking for a new friend too.

JUST ONE WEEK INTO MY NEW JOB AT THE RADIO STATION, I'm given my biggest interview yet.

Freddie has arranged for me to interview Umukuka Wilson Wamimbi, the newly elected king of Masaaba. It is a win-win situation for both of us: Freddie's station is proud to boast an American journalist. And I am on a king's porch, notebook in hand, just a couple of days before his official coronation.

The home is modest but well crafted. A lanky and quick assistant pours hot tea into squat mugs, then steps away to wait under the shade of a tree.

While Uganda is primarily led by a president, there are kings who preside over each cultural region and preserve the traditions of the tribes. I have been staying in the Bamasaaba territory, which includes more than 5.5 million people in an area that extends from Eastern Uganda into Western Kenya.

We settle back onto a bench on the patio of his country home, located among the sprawling coffee plantations on the outskirts of Mbale. He is dressed in a marine blue button-down shirt and a pair of khakis that look freshly laundered and pressed. His face is friendly, pleated with deep lines across his forehead. He folds his hands and waits for me to speak.

"Okay," I say, taking a deep breath before I launch into some warm-up questions. Then I ask if he's always wanted to be king.

Wamimbi is reserved and insists that I call him a "traditional leader" rather than "king."

"No. I never expected anything like this," he says. "To be given the responsibility of leading people is a great honor. It is like becoming the mother of a large family."

The job of a cultural king is an important one; Uganda is a country that clings to the past while striding into the future, a place where witch doctors have offices next to medical clinics. We have a long discussion about finding the delicate balance between those worlds, moving both of them forward together.

After about an hour of conversation, I have one last question.

"If you're a king, will you wear a crown?" I ask.

"Only for very special occasions," he laughs.

At his coronation a few days later, he does indeed don a crown, a tall cone stitched in leather and covered in pale cowry shells. Police in olive-colored uniforms patrol the gate of the wooden fence that lines the perimeter of the grounds of the celebration area. Those with invitations, including me, are welcomed inside to sit on plastic chairs under fabric circus tents. Those without invitations wedge themselves along the fence.

Wamimbi's plain gray suit is covered by a shield made of animal skin to symbolize that he is the protector of his people. He also carries a spear to demonstrate his power. The crowd is silent as he makes vows of unity and promises to be a fair and kind leader.

During his speech, which is given in both English and Swahili, the two official languages of Uganda, Wamimbi stresses the importance of preserving cultural heritage.

"We've already lost too much of our traditions over time, so I will focus on restoring and preserving those," he says. "Without our culture, we are nothing."

This celebratory site is also home to another traditional Bamasaaba event—the male circumcision ritual, called *imbalu*, which takes place every other year during a three-day festival. As many as 40,000 teenage boys, smeared in a yeast-like porridge, receive their initiation into manhood from a traditional healer while the villagers dance and cheer.

That is acknowledged by one of the clan elders as he glances around the throng of thousands at the king's coronation.

"Impressive crowd," I say. "Many people."

He leans over and whispers, "The circumcisions draw a bigger crowd."

Now a tide of clan elders and dancers ebb and flow around Wamimbi as he circles the cultural grounds. Feet and homemade drums thunder like thousands of hooves pounding across the red dirt. Whooping noises shatter the thick, humid air.

I feel like part of a blended tribe myself, and the cultural display forces me to think about my heritage. I try to imagine what it must have been like for my mother when she married my father, the leap she made for love. She barely spoke English, and she had never traveled beyond Europe. As soon as they were wed, my dad was stationed to an air force base in New Mexico. Such a stark difference from the place where she grew up.

My mom quickly became pregnant with my older sister, but my dad's work kept him busy, leaving her alone in a place she didn't understand. It was a sparse landscape populated by dust storms and scrub brush. The open sky must have felt so isolating. She once told me she cried after every appointment with her obstetrician, because so much was happening with her body and she didn't know how to communicate it.

My sister, Monica, was born in 1963. My brother, Mark, came along two years later. Then my dad was deployed to Vietnam for a year. He wrote letters to my mother every single day, an extended, one-sided conversation about sticky jungles and mess hall spaghetti. It's hard for me to imagine how she navigated her loneliness, stuck in the arid land with two children, unable to drive, barely able to communicate.

I came along many years later, when my family was stationed in Georgia. There are thirteen years between my sister and me, eleven years' difference with my brother. By that time, my mother's English was impeccable. When she showed up at the hospital in labor to have me, she was initially turned away. There were no rooms. She was given the address of the bigger hospital across town and told to go there.

"I am having this baby, and I am having it here," she said.

That is why I was born in a linen closet. Because my mom insisted on staying, and she was too much of a force to be reckoned with.

In Uganda I watch a group of younger dancers swirl into the mass of drummers and warriors. Their skirts are long and indigo, their white shirts untucked. Their belts and headbands look like strips of bark. They chant and holler, calling out the new king's full title. The songs they perform tell stories of struggle, then triumph over trauma.

I let my mind wander back to when I was in my early twenties and learned about the other sibling. The one without a name.

This happened while I was living in a small town in Appalachia, about one year after my mom's diagnosis. My dad asked me to come home for the weekend to take care of mom so he could attend his high school reunion in Indiana.

Though my mom was in the early stages of Alzheimer's, the disease was pronounced enough that she couldn't be left alone. She could eat, dress herself, and use the toilet without any assistance, but she had to be told to do those things. A bold red stop sign posted on the inside of the front door reminded her that she shouldn't leave the house. Her wrist was outfitted with an electronic bracelet that could be tracked by the sheriff's department, in case she decided to wander anyway.

I didn't want to go home that weekend, even though my dad needed my help. I was twenty-four and awful. It was a challenge for me to find compassion; I had a lot of anger. I resented the disease that had replaced my mom with somebody foreign. I felt like I had been abandoned by her and given only the memory of a woman. She had begun to smell acrid and old, like stale flowers and ammonia and lemon drops. I missed her perfume, the sharp one I once hated. Her new body revolted me, so pale and unfamiliar. I couldn't bear to be around her.

How sad it is to know your mom for only twenty-four years. I was only just beginning to be a person. I needed her.

My life in those days was one poor choice after another and a readiness to escape my reality. I drank a lot, to the point where I thought it was normal to start every day by dry heaving. I was secretly dating a local politician and spent my weekends having sex with him in the back of the minivan he shared with his recently separated wife. My needs were simple, and I was easily fulfilled: I wanted to see him and fall asleep to a dizzy ceiling and forget my life. The last place I wanted to go was home.

I reluctantly agreed to take care of my mom anyway. That weekend, looking for a way to waste time, I brought her to a bookstore.

My mom was excruciatingly slow getting out of the car. I unbuckled her seat belt and helped her stand up. She took tiny steps across the parking lot. In front of the door, she snapped to a halt. People pushed by, grumbled. I was embarrassed. My mom turned to me and her eyes searched mine. It had been months since she had looked at my face like this, with some kind of recognition. It felt real, and it made me want to cry.

"There's something you should know," she said. She rocked her weight to her right foot, which meant she was completely blocking the door now. I tugged on her arm and pulled her to the side. She winced.

"There's something you should know," she said again, this time with greater urgency.

I sighed. "What is it, Mom?" I was irritated. I wanted to get inside this bookstore, where people wouldn't stare at us.

She furrowed her brow. "You have another brother," she said.

I sighed. How many other things had she created in her mind? The disease eating away at her brain manifested some mighty fantasies. She thought there was a pattern in the red cars that passed by the house. She thought the planes overhead, landing at the nearby air force base, were sending signals to my father. She imagined the rooftops of our neighbors' houses were used to communicate a secret code that somehow was being used by my father to get away with an elaborate affair. None of this was true.

Now I had another brother. Yeah, right.

I held my mother's hand and walked her inside the bookstore. I sat her down in the section closest to the door. I did my best to collect myself, to be patient. This disease wasn't her fault.

"Mom, I know you think I have another brother," I said. "But you have a disease called Alzheimer's."

She looked at me with pity then, as if I were some kind of rube. She reached for her purse but couldn't unzip it. I helped her open the bag. She retrieved her wallet, which she also couldn't open. Again, I helped. The wallet was a mess of faded receipts, phone numbers, expired credit cards. She hadn't used it in at least a couple of years, but she carried it out of habit.

Behind all the pockets and clear sleeves of photos, there was a secret compartment, where she used to hide layaway receipts for the clothes and purses she bought without telling my dad. From that compartment, she pulled out a tiny black-and-white photo.

It was a boy. Light hair and light eyes, just like my mom. Her distinctive, sloping nose. Same face shape. So familiar, and yet it was a boy I had never seen before.

"This is your other brother," she said.

It made no sense. How could this boy look so much like my mom?

The words came quickly: "I was raped. I got pregnant. I gave the boy away, and he was adopted by an American family. This is the only photo I have. This is all I have. This is my boy."

"That is not your boy," I said. My brother Mark was her boy, not that light-haired kid. We weren't a family with dark, unexplored closets and things left unsaid. My mother and I didn't keep secrets.

"This is my boy," she murmured again.

The people around us didn't seem to notice that my family had just splintered. Shoppers plucked books from the shelves. A teenage girl gestured dramatically to her friend with a cup of Starbucks. I heard the ding of the cash register.

Then my mom was gone again, like someone snuffed out a candle. Her eyes dimmed. Her shoulders slumped. She looked down at her wallet with disdain, like it was a crumpled tissue someone had just dropped into her lap. This is what happened sometimes in this stage of the disease—a snap of clarity before she drooped back into the fog—though these moments had become more rare. I barely got to see my real mom anymore.

I folded up the wallet and snapped it shut, put it back in the purse. I couldn't accept this—that the woman I thought I knew so well was never known to me at all; that her secret compartments held much more than a receipt for an expensive skirt.

I have always been one of three children. Now I am one of four? I never considered this piece of my identity to be malleable.

"Let's go," I said, and I held her arm as I guided her away from the store.

Later that night at my parents' home, I repeated everything to my dad while I made a pot of decaf in the kitchen.

"It was so crazy," I said. "She said I have another brother. Can you believe that?"

"Well, you do," he said.

His tone was straightforward. Terse. I told him I didn't understand.

"Your mother never wanted you to think she was tainted," my dad said. "She never wanted you to know she suffered. She was too strong for that."

I always knew she was strong. I just never imagined how resilient. For so many years, my mom never revealed the story to my siblings or me, not until the flash at the bookstore, when that ancient, hungry pain cracked her open and broke through.

After learning that, I decided I couldn't let my mom's disease make me a worse person. She would want me to be stronger than that. So I made a list of things I wanted: a new job, accomplishments outside of the bar, a boyfriend I didn't have to keep secret. It took a little while, but I set my life on a new course. I found, through her struggle, a new path for myself.

In Uganda on a crushing hot day, I watch the warriors dance around Umukuka Wilson Wamimbi. Their feathers tremble with their movements as they dance a story about the clan's history. They create the narrative for their tribe, and they define how they are seen in the world. Their cries sound deep and familiar, the sound of longing, the sound of loss, the sound of unity, the sound of a clan.

I understand that sound. My mother is a warrior too.

You Can Survive the Bad Place

⬿⬿⬿

AFTER MBALE, I RETURN TO KAMPALA FOR A FEW DAYS BE-
fore the city begins to wear on me and I hop on a bus for my next adventure.

It takes more than two hours to fully escape the frenetic crowds and wild streets of Kampala. Finally we reach a point where the asphalt is exhausted, becoming firmly packed roads of red clay. Dense, shoulder-to-shoulder buildings disappear, replaced by green trees and modest houses. Each time the bus shudders to a stop, hawkers run to the windows selling skewers of meat, bags of fruit, or warm chapati bread rolled around a thin egg omelet, what they call a "Rolex."

Men zip through the streets on motorbikes, bare-chested, not slowed at all by the long yellow kayaks that balance perpendicularly across the backs of their bikes. When I see them, that's how I know we've reached Jinja, a bucolic town that has become East Africa's hub for adventure sports. People from all over the world travel here for the world-class kayaking, the all-terrain vehicle safaris, and the epic bungee jumping. I'm here to go whitewater rafting at the source of the Nile River.

My backpacker hostel is situated on a hill that overlooks sinuous curves of water. This is where the tour company will pick us up in the morning. I'm staying in a dorm room with several other adventure seekers, all more experienced than I am. I've never been whitewater rafting, but my favorite amusement park ride as a kid was White Water Canyon at Kings Island in Mason, Ohio, and for some reason, I imagine this real-life experience will be essentially the same thing: a refreshing float on some burbling water through woodland scenery, a height requirement of at least forty-six inches, possibly a funnel cake afterward.

As the sun sets, I open a cold Tusker lager and carefully read the waiver for the next day's rafting trip. The paper says the rapids in Jinja are "grade five on a scale that runs from one to six." Grade one means mild rocking and rolling, suitable for beginners. Grade six presents extreme danger and barely navigable rapids, even for professionals.

So. Grade five? Holy mother of paddling. This requires skillful maneuvering of choppy water, huge hazards, steep drops, and crashing waves. It also means that as a first-timer, I am terrified. The chapati bread I ate on arrival now churns uncomfortably in my stomach. My throat burns and tastes acidic. I knew the rapids were a five before I signed up—I just thought the scale ran from one to ten.

That night I call Jason via Skype. When he answers, I tell him what I'm about to do. I expect him to be proud of me.

"So this might be goodbye," I laugh.

"Then why are you doing this?" he snaps. He's angry, so different from the man who held my hand on a skydiving aircraft during the ride to altitude and told me to relax in the sky. "Nobody's forcing you to go rafting."

"People always say that when you grow old, you'll regret the things you didn't do, not the things you did."

"That's *if* you grow old," he replies.

It's a joke, but the rest of the conversation is strained. I wish I knew how to comfort him, but it's hard to do over a jumpy internet connection, especially when I am equally apprehensive.

I think about my mother in her quiet room at the nursing home. She was proud to be a mostly stay-at-home mom while I was growing up, and she worked hard to create a safe, warm environment there. After she became ill, my dad retired from the air force, determined to keep her at home for as long as he could. He really tried.

Eventually my mom forgot how to go to the bathroom; sometimes she used the sink, sometimes the bathtub, and that's when she wasn't fighting the process altogether. She forgot how to eat; sometimes her mouth was mid-bite when she forgot that she needed to chew the food. In the middle of the night, she was restless and unsettled and often woke in a panic. She forgot the identity of the man sleeping next to her; that's when she became violent. My dad considered buying a gun, just for his own safety.

My dad was devastated the day he signed my mom over to the nursing home and drove home alone. But she required a level of care he could no longer give.

The remainder of her life will be spent in one hushed and sterile room, a thought that always leaves me cold and afraid. I know she'd rather be facing rapids than losing more of herself each day. I know she would take chances if she had the opportunity. I have to do this, because she cannot.

I sign the waiver.

The next morning, twenty of us are taken by bus from the hostel to the launch point. My heart is pounding so hard I hardly hear the employee who asks for my payment. In return for fifty dollars, I'm handed a long paddle. I have no idea how to hold it, even on steady ground. The paddle is awkward and cumbersome, like I've been gifted a third arm.

Here at the launch point, the Nile River is jagged, a silver expanse that slices through the morning mist. I slip my toes into the river, the longest in the world. The water I see now will flow north from this point all the way to the Mediterranean Sea, a journey of three months and 6,800 kilometers.

From the dock, the rafts look as tiny as poppy seeds floating in an Olympic-sized pool. My raft of five other people, all strangers to me, is the last to launch into the river.

Our captain is Jane, a long-limbed, muscular blonde with hair braided into taut cornrows that reveal tanned strips of scalp. Her Australian accent gives the impression of someone who guzzles stocky cans of Foster's beer and wrestles crocodiles, which is soothing since there are, indeed, crocodiles around us.

Jane barks, "Wild or mild?"

Our group is divided. Half want the more aggressive experience, while the others want something more subdued. Jane narrows her eyes and shakes her head with disapproval. She looks feral, and I'm certain we're in store for something fierce.

Despite my fear, I feel completely present in this moment. The air is hot and stagnant, and the rubbery smell coming from the red raft is strong and medicinal. The shore appears far and unreachable, like a distant mirage on the horizon. Insects skim the Nile with grace.

Jane teaches us how to hold the paddle and scoop the water, propelling us forward. She chastises me for not digging deep, merely skimming the surface. After ten minutes of calm, placid rafting, Jane abruptly—and deliberately—tips the boat, forcing us to swim through a set of small, milky rapids.

I am plunged into both the river and the memory of the last time I was overpowered by water. My mother never learned to swim, and she wanted me to seize every opportunity she never had. So I dutifully attended classes at the Dayton YMCA, even while I maintained a weak stroke and a strong fear of drowning, dog-paddling my way through each level: polliwog, guppy, minnow, fish. Up I climbed through the aquatic food chain. When I somehow attained shark, I was tested on my ability to tread water while fully clothed. The goal was to last a half hour in the deep section of the pool, and toward the end I gave out. My memory of it is more like a montage of film clips—sinking, inhaling water, struggling to the surface, coughing, chlorine tears burning my cheeks, and my mom on the side of the pool, howling for help. She looked beautiful even in her panic, her short, curly blonde hair teased around her head, her poppy lips frozen into an O. I don't remember a single thing she said, only that she looked perfect while I flailed.

Now, here in Eastern Uganda, it is baptism by boulders. I emerge on the other side of the rocks bruised and with a stomach full of Nile water. I bob to the surface, white-knuckling my life jacket. I'm okay, but I'm irritated. I've put myself in the hands of this Jane woman, and she didn't think twice about tossing me from the boat.

After the raft is righted, I hoist myself into it again. Jane gives our group the option to bail out now and float down another part of the river in a safety boat instead of tackling any more rapids. *Go, fool, go!* yells the sane part of my brain. But I can't. If I turn back now, I'll always doubt myself. I'll forever be the eleven-year-old girl, sinking in the deep end at the Y in Dayton.

It's a shock when I discover the first few rapids are actually fun. Each time we approach rocks and roaring water, Jane cries, "Paddle-paddle-paddle!" followed by a quick "Get down!" We dutifully obey her commands. Our raft successfully skims rapids and slides down waterfalls.

We reach a treacherous spot known as Itanda, "the bad place," a series of rapids in quick succession. I dig my paddle in—Jane would be proud if she were paying attention—but the raft spirals as though we're not even tending to it. As I heave and grunt, I peek at the other people in my boat and see we're all grappling with this thing. I see the sturdy, brute determination to survive.

At the other side, I'm surprised to find myself still aloft. We've made it through.

Then we meet the rapids called Silverback, a name Jane speaks with reverence. I know we're in for it. I can hear it coming. The green river churns and crashes against pointed rocks like a terrible, bubbling stew. I close my eyes. I don't want to see what's coming.

I think about my last visit home before leaving on my backpacking trip. My dad brought me to the nursing home, and we entered the elevator. He knew the security code to make the doors close—this is a safety feature to prevent the Alzheimer's patients from wandering onto another floor or out of the building. My dad paused.

"You might not recognize your mother anymore—the disease has taken a real physical toll in the past few months," he said. I braced myself for the worst, my stomach hard with dread.

When the elevator opened, my dad gestured across the room.

"There she is."

I forced my eyes to open, and I saw the skeleton of a woman arranged on a recliner. Her eyes were sunken, and her cheeks were two dark hollows. I gasped.

"No, no, no," I cried, the words rushing forth before I could stop them.

The waves swallow the boat whole, and I'm still not looking. In an instant I feel the raft drop out from under me, and I am airborne for a brief moment before I am chewed by raging water.

"That's not your mother," my dad said gently. "Look behind her."

She wore no makeup, and her hair was gray and limp. Her shirt was nothing pretty, and the elastic band of her pants was pulled up far too high. But there was no doubt. This was my mother, the woman who birthed me, who nurtured me, who challenged me to become everything she couldn't. She didn't know me enough to love me anymore, but every part of me remembered her.

My head barely breaks the surface before the swells hammer me again. When I open my mouth, it is partially underwater, partially above. I inhale a mixture of sweet air and frothy, murky foam. Above there's muck and dirt and a kaleidoscopic shimmer of waves.

Sour river water slides through my nose, cutting a raw path down my throat. I splash around and somehow my right hand makes contact with the raft. My shoulder feels hot and heavy as I grab the rope and cling to it.

My arm is fiercely yanked one way. More rapids. In the chaos of rocks and waves, the raft is torn from my grasp. *Crocodiles*, I think. *Oh my God, what about the fucking crocodiles?* I curl into a ball, some kind of animal instinct, and then I am rolling, tumbling downstream, whisked through a channel of noise and turbulence, the container inside a pneumatic tube. If the crocs are nearby, I'm surely moving too fast for any of them to catch me. When my head breaks the surface again, I don't know how much time or distance has passed. But the water is calm, the boat is gone, and I am alone.

I wipe water from my eyes and float for a few minutes looking up at the sky, the river holding me like a soft hand, before a safety kayak glides toward me and tows me to a larger safety boat. After I hoist myself inside, I cough, but not productively. I try to summon enough muscle to bark out the water in my lungs.

A paddle bobs on the surface nearby, and I heave it into the boat with me. Several minutes later, my sinuses clear. My ears pop. I finally catch my breath. My heartbeat slows to a normal rate. And it's a relief when more heads bob up nearby—the rest of my group. They swim to the safety boat, and I help tug them inside. Only one girl is bloody, but her cuts are shallow, and our nervous conversation gives way to excited hugs. We are all okay, and the river has offered us solidarity. Swapping stories about our rapids, adrenaline flowing like a geyser, we don't feel much like strangers anymore.

When Jane appears, unscathed, from an inlet with our boat, we all cheer. I'm one of the first to leap into the water and swim to the raft, and I'm genuinely happy to be back in it. We drift for about an hour on a placid portion of river. Jane hands me an orange, and I drop the peel into the water. It curls and floats lazily for a moment, until it catches a current and is torn away. I imagine it gliding from here through the newly formed country of South Sudan, mingling with sediment from the Blue Nile and White Nile tributaries, sweeping past Egypt's farmlands and tombs, washing ashore somewhere in the Mediterranean. Maybe somebody will find this proof of my existence and wonder where it came from.

When I was still an active skydiver, I kept a letter in my desk to be given to my family in the event of the worst-case scenario. The letter explained how my life was richer for them being a part of it, and I offered assurance that I wanted it to end this way—though risky, I believed that death while soaring was both noble and true. But I didn't write any letters before I left for this trip. I realize now it's because I expect to survive. I've hauled my way through the bad place, and I'm traveling the route that will bring me home again.

My legs are tired and my skin is sunburned. When I look to the horizon, I see churning water. It's time to paddle. I sit erect in the boat, and I stare down the whirlpools and rocks. When the waves strike, I refuse to close my eyes. This time I approach them on my own terms. The raft remains steady.

For the last few rapids, I don't even need to hear Jane's instructions to know what to do. Our boat never capsizes again, and my group successfully finishes twenty-five kilometers from where we began.

It's early evening when I jump from the raft for the last time. The sun sinks behind the tangle of scruffy trees, and the river is broad and black, open as a wound. The air has cooled considerably, and the water is chilly. I keep my limbs warm with a few freestyle strokes, making shimmery waves with each movement. My new friends call from the muddy bank, but I'm not ready to head for shore yet.

I remember from school that the Nile is shaped like the lotus flower, a symbol of renewal for the ancient Egyptians. Right now I am in the stem, pulling myself toward the blossom.

Some Things Can't Be Understood, Only Experienced

───⊗⊗⊗───

A REGGAE-THEMED HOSTEL IN KIGALI, RWANDA, SOUNDED so promising in the guidebook: "If it's the spirit of peace and harmony you are after, then this little retreat is the place for you."

Peace? Harmony? Retreat? I didn't even need to read about any other lodgings. This one sounded perfect.

Upon arrival, I'm surprised to discover this retreat is surrounded by a concrete fence, a massive metal gate, and a guard post at the entrance. The gardens are overgrown. The office is a small room with a cashbox on a table and skinny yellow cats that zigzag around my ankles. Aged posters of Bob Marley hang on the wall.

Near the guesthouse where I'll be staying is a prosthetic workshop, where limbs are made for people who lost theirs during the 1994 genocide. Stray wooden limbs clutter the paths to the rooms, and some of them are broken.

I didn't exchange any money at the border—the exchange rate was incredibly poor—so I arrived in the country with a pocket full of now-useless Ugandan shillings and some emergency American bills. The hostel clerk says he will accept the U.S. money, but only if I pay for a three-night stay at a higher-than-usual exchange rate. Tired and desperate, I fork over the money. I don't even ask to see the room.

I unlock my room and see that I'm paying thirty-five dollars a night for what feels like a tall jail cell. Though Rwanda is known as "the land of one thousand hills," I won't be able to see any of them from here, even when it is light outside—the cinder-block walls loom cold and hard, about fifteen feet high, with just one small window near the ceiling. The room is not much more than a square of gray with a bed and one chair.

A low stone wall partitions off a private bathroom that consists of a shower head, a clogged drain, and a toilet that doesn't flush. The water in the pipes runs cold and colder. For an extra ten dollars a night, I could have received an "upgrade"—that is, the owner would turn on the hot water. I can't afford that kind of luxury on my budget. Or food, for that matter.

I scrounge around in a red nylon bag that I keep packed with assorted foodstuffs. My dinner choices include a box of pasta, a packet of powdered pumpkin soup, two packets of maple syrup–flavored instant oatmeal, a bag of peppermint tea, and a three-month-old smashed granola bar from Bolivia.

Since most of those items require hot water, I go with the Bolivian granola. It is not good, unless you enjoy sawdust with raisins, but it quiets my growling stomach.

Mosquitoes swarm the room, and I huddle under the net that hangs over my bed. It is dusty pink, and it looks like it has been belched out from the ceiling, chunky, saggy, and full of knots. It has big rips that I try to fix with duct tape. Some of the bugs still manage to find a way in. I hear them buzzing around my head, echoing in my ears.

I'm not even sure what I'm doing in Rwanda, except seeking a new place to volunteer. The country seemed manageable, since the whole nation is just slightly smaller than the state of Maryland. It helped that it was an incredibly easy border jump from Kampala to Kigali. The bus journey took just eight hours, which is lightning speed in African bus time, and cost the equivalent of ten dollars.

Only now that I'm here, I'm not sure what to do. This night seems darker than most, and I hunker down on the bed with a book. I long for my husband's voice, but I have no cell service or internet access, and he has no way of knowing where in the world I am.

The room's one light dangles from the ceiling with exposed wires. I'm not even surprised when it extinguishes itself, as if it has committed suicide. *I'm with you, light. I give up too.*

So I cry. I cry as the room remains frustratingly dark. I cry as mosquitoes zoom into my ears. I cry as the toilet spontaneously hiccups fetid water onto the floor of the bathroom. And then I cry deeper, a heavy sob of guilt, knowing that I'm in a land that has faced genocide and unspeakable horror. I cry for the people I've never known and the people I never will know and the ache of things I cannot possibly understand. I cry for a mom who is dying while I am unable to stop it and for all the incomplete families that surround me.

That night I dream of malaria and detached body parts. Though I sleep, it feels more like a pause than rest.

When morning arrives, I am thankful to open up the door and see that the sun has come up. Prosthetic legs still litter the ground, but now I won't trip over them.

BY THE END OF MY FIRST FULL DAY IN KIGALI, I HAVE Rwandan francs in my pocket and a belly full of sweet potatoes, beans, and cassava from a local mélange, or buffet. Still I feel aimless and lonely.

I settle into an internet café and spend a couple of hours searching for a place to volunteer. My one lead—I had traded emails about teaching at a women's shelter with one of the organization's administrators—ends when what they need is clarified: "Can you teach aerobics? In French?" I thought they wanted a writing instructor.

Before heading back to the dreaded hostel, I take a walk through downtown Kigali. It's more residential than I'd imagined. The houses are big and stately, made of solid brick, the windows lined with flower boxes. The streets are leafy and clean, the lawns trim and decisively green. It's as hard to imagine a genocide taking place here as it would be on my street of palm trees and bougainvillea in Palm Springs. I continue walking, knowing that people died on the ground where my feet are now.

The genocide began after years of tension between Hutus and Tutsis. The fire ignited on April 6, 1994, when the plane carrying Rwandan president Juvénal Habyarimana was shot down as it prepared to land in Kigali.

Violence moved swiftly throughout the tiny country. The quickness and efficiency of it was astonishing—one person killed every seven seconds. Print and radio media added more fuel to the fire with violent propaganda, encouraging war rape and urging the Hutu people to exterminate their "cockroach" Tutsi neighbors.

Roads were closed, trapping people inside their towns and villages. Those who sought refuge in churches were betrayed and slaughtered there instead. Family members turned on their loved ones with machetes. There are stories that those who attempted to flee had their Achilles tendons sliced, so they were forced to witness the bloodbath that surrounded them before they were bludgeoned to death.

By the time the massacre ended in mid-July 1994, just one hundred days later, every tenth person was dead—a significant chunk of a country with a population equivalent to that of Chicago. More than 500,000 others were mutilated. Many had been raped and infected with HIV.

There is nothing I can do but let the sadness burrow inside me. What else can be done when surrounded by so many ghosts?

DAYS PASS. I MOVE OUT OF THE PROSTHETIC-LIMB FACTORY and into a youth hostel that is closer to downtown. The building is spacious and crayon yellow, full of long-term backpackers, graduate students who are living in Rwanda to study the genocide, and expatriates who work for nongovernment organizations. At night we sit on the patio and drink big, cold bottles of Primus beer and rarely discuss the tragedy that happened in this place.

My new neighborhood is where the president lives, a posh section of the city filled with wide streets, flower beds, and embassies. Snipers line the nearby rooftops. It becomes such a commonplace sight that I don't even notice them after my first day at the hostel.

In addition to a place to live, I also find a reason to be in Rwanda, as a volunteer in a trade school for adult women. All of them either lost their families or encountered other troubles after the genocide, which then led them to prostitution. Now they come to this school to learn skills like jewelry making, weaving, and sewing. My job is to teach them practical English, just enough phrases to help them tell their stories and sell their homemade goods to tourists.

To get to the school, I take a *moto* taxi (what Ugandans called a boda-boda), showing up the same time every weekday afternoon. About 75 percent of the time, Andre the guard opens the metal gate to let me inside. The other 25 percent of the time, Andre is huddled in his room with Francois the cook, watching soap operas on a tiny black-and-white TV. On those days I shout until a student hears me and unlocks the maroon metal door.

My class consists of twenty-five students, give or take. Mostly take. They are not required to be there, so I usually end up with about twelve people. Even the students who say they are excited to learn English slouch in their metal chairs and roll their eyes.

I start by teaching general phrases and introductions: "Hello" and "good morning." "How are you?" and "What is your name?"

Evoking classroom participation is practically impossible—I beg the students to answer my questions or repeat after me. I have never been a teacher before, and filling up an hour of instruction every afternoon is excruciating.

When I remind myself that I'm not certified for this, it makes me feel more selfish than kindhearted. I have no background in education—I'm just trying to pass along some of my knowledge about the English language. I wonder how much good I'm doing. Why should I ask these students to call me "teacher" when I am not one? What if my volunteer work harms these women? What if I'm taking a position away from someone more qualified to help?

After the first few days, I bring my concerns to Tom, the administrator who initially interviewed me, and I ask him if I should abandon the volunteer post. He is a British man who has been helping to run this school and nonprofit for more than a dozen years. During that time, he has seen many volunteers come and go, and he has seen how the school prepares the women for practical jobs in modern Rwanda.

"Listen, you are important," he says. "If they didn't care about your lessons, they wouldn't come to your class."

But the next day, toward the end of my fifth class, I wonder again. Liberé, the slouchiest one of them all, swipes chalk dust off the board and pats my back, leaving stark white handprints on my black T-shirt. The other students hoot and cackle at me while they applaud Liberé. It's just a silly joke, probably made with no malicious intent, but it makes me feel disliked, unwanted, marked. I see who has the power here in this room, and it's not the woman standing at the front of the class. My face grows hot and red, and I leave quickly, before I break down in front of everybody.

Back at the hostel, my roommates are already pumping music and getting ready for the weekend. But they won't see me at the clubs; I'm going to find a way to win over my classroom.

I spend hours researching how to teach English as a second language, how to capture a classroom's attention, and how to create a useful and practical learning experience for them. Selfishly, what I want is for my class to like me. I want them to accept me. This is high school all over again.

The next Monday, I try out a trick I remember from my own teachers: I bribe the class with candy. One wrapped caramel for each answer. Suddenly I can barely keep up with their enthusiasm.

By the time I ask "Which direction am I pointing?" a dozen hands shoot up in the air. I shuffle the tables and chairs around the room until I have created a labyrinth that leads to the front of the room. Then I blindfold myself. I ask the students to guide me through the complicated maze by using their new direction words. When someone says "left" instead of "right," I let myself walk into walls or stumble into a desk—I already feel stupid enough in front of my class that I might as well look like it too. In response, the students laugh and scream with delight. A few of them yell "No!" and try to stop me from tumbling over a chair.

That day, everybody gets candy. And I get my first invitation to hang out with a couple of students outside of the classroom: Rose and Claudine ask me to go for a walk in their neighborhood. I am elated as they steer me down the brown path to their homes.

TWO WEEKS INTO TEACHING, AND I'VE LEARNED THAT EV-erything in Rwanda requires a follow-up question. I discover this during my lesson about families, as I teach vocabulary words like "sister," "father," "husband."

When I pose the question "Do you have brothers and sisters?" to my students, I am met with stares until I follow that with "*Did* you have brothers and sisters?" That's when I begin to hear their stories. Time is separated into pre- and post-genocide, and so are the tenses in which my students ask me to speak.

I can't even fathom this pain. I spend each day surrounded by women my age who have fought to survive. They outlasted a genocide while I was selecting dyed-to-match shoes for prom. They saw hatred and destruction firsthand. Me, I watched danger on TV. They watched loved ones die from machete blows. I'm grieving a mother who rests in a clean nursing home bed.

The genocide is like a man lurking in the shadows, a faceless stranger who feels present even when he is not. This affects every conversation, every interaction. It changes how people look at each other, how they appraise strangers, how guarded they remain.

Claudine and I walk the neighborhood after class one day, and she tells me her story. When her Hutu neighbors came for her Tutsi family, she hid underneath her bed while they beat her father until he was unable to move. A neighbor dragged Claudine into the room and handed her the machete. Only sixteen years old, she was forced to make the final blow.

When Claudine tried to run, the same machete was used to slice her legs, and some of the men beat her with sticks. They laughed as she crawled for help. That's when she blacked out. She doesn't remember what happened next or how she survived. But she does know that when the genocide began, she was an HIV-free teenager with a family. By the time it ended, she was an HIV-positive woman, alone.

I struggle to understand an event that breaks the brittle bones of what I once believed to be true: people are inherently good, and sometimes the world just makes them do bad things. The reality in Rwanda is that evil exists, and my students have borne witness.

Beyond that, I wonder if this is even my tragedy to understand. The struggle of my own mortality feels selfish in the face of those trying to reconcile their humanity, and I have no right to stake a claim in their personal suffering. I can't escape the fact that I am a foreigner here, and I always will be. I can grieve here, but what right do I have to feel so sad?

I remember what Jason said about how the brain tries to compartmentalize anything it doesn't already understand, how our minds try to find patterns in clouds. I think about the genocide, but it dissipates in front of me. My brain tries to make sense of the senseless, and I see nothing familiar there at all.

There Is No Hierarchy of Pain

I DON'T KNOW WHY I DECIDE TO VISIT SEVERAL GENOCIDE
memorials. Maybe it's that I want to understand my students' stories better.
Maybe I need to mourn for a mother other than my own.

I make the trip to Murambi alone and by bus. Once there, it is an easy
walk to the school.

I'm close to the school complex when my step slows. My walk has started
to sound like an autumn hike through the forest, with sticks popping and
cracking on the path beneath my feet. But when I look around, I notice there
aren't many trees nearby. The landscape is flat and grassy. There shouldn't be
sticks underfoot.

When I squat down, the dirt is embedded with tiny bones. I hold some
of them in my hands; they are small and light, almost like bird skeletons.
A volunteer, who had been standing on the school porch, walks toward me,
crossing the grass until she is close enough that her shadow stretches over
mine.

"Kids," she says.

I let the bones fall from my hands, returning them to their exposed grave. I don't know what else to do with them.

Most of the school buildings before me are plain and low-slung like barracks. It's here that thousands of Tutsis were instructed by government officials to seek sanctuary. The whole idea of a sanctuary was a ruse—the officials deliberately gathered the Tutsis in one place, denied them water and food, then slaughtered everyone when they were too weak to escape. An estimated 45,000 live here now, in this earth.

The volunteer, a genocide survivor, opens the door of the school and ushers me inside. I've seen a few dead bodies in my life. While working the nighttime crime beat at the *Cincinnati Enquirer*, I saw glimpses of death—limbs askew under white sheets, puddles of blood, the silhouette of a body as it is rolled away—but now I am in a room with hundreds of dead at once.

There are wooden tables in every classroom, each covered with children and adults, who were initially buried in mass graves then exhumed, now calcified white from powdered lime. Their shapes are contorted, twisted, and frozen in the moment of death. Some of the bodies look more like papier-mâché than people. Others looks like crumpled sheets.

Each rigid limb tells a story. Even though the skin of each person has long since shriveled, on a few, the machete slashes are plainly visible. Some fingers still bear wedding rings. Mothers cradle the void. Hands grip the air. Mouths are forever wide in silent screams.

The lime is supposed to absorb odors, but it is not strong enough to mask what has happened here. With every inhale, my nose fills with the scent of decay, and my stomach lurches in revulsion. I am angry and sorrowful, underscored by guilt.

Until my mom was diagnosed with Alzheimer's, I lived with the assumption of a future. Even now, I am resentful of the genetics I might carry and how this holds the rest of my life captive, because I believe I am entitled to one. The bodies that surround me didn't have that luxury. They were promised a future, and it was a lie.

I know it's better to show the bones of victims instead of hiding them, but that doesn't make it easier to see. I rush through the remaining twenty-three rooms, all filled with bodies, until the final hall, a place of meditation and prayer. I sit on a bench for a long time—long enough for the guide to peek her head into the room and make certain I'm all right. I want to be alone, so I wave her away, but she stays with me anyway.

ANOTHER DAY, ANOTHER BUS, THIS TIME HEADED AN HOUR south of Kigali to Nyamata, site of another memorial. Our bus slips along the hilly highway, tires tearing across the washboard shoulders, sliding toward drop-off cliffs, then back on the asphalt again. Luckily, the road is nearly empty.

The man sitting next to me drops his head between his knees and groans. In his right hand he clutches a lime, digging his fingernails into the puckered skin. Every few minutes he holds the lime to his nose and inhales, the punchy scent smoothing over his motion sickness.

"My stomach tumbles," he says, moaning with discomfort.

Mine does too, but not from the bus ride. Death is everywhere, and no amount of citrus zest will fix the way I feel.

On my regular calls home, my dad hasn't said much about my mom's health, even when I ask. It makes me wonder what he's keeping from me. I know she has spent the past few months in the "moderately severe" stage of Alzheimer's. She has little awareness of her surroundings; she rarely responds to her own name; she needs help eating, dressing, and going to the toilet; and she no longer walks. I also know that once my mom reaches the final stage—when she becomes completely unresponsive—it won't be long until her body shuts down entirely.

We reach the small town of Nyamata. The moment I step off the bus, a handful of touts crowd around me, all shouting. "Miss, I take you to genocide church! Fair price!" "Lady, you want to see big grave?" I push through the crowd, the men scatter, and I am alone again.

I walk through the town and up a hillside to the place where the ghosts live. The church.

When the genocide began, many of Nyamata's residents took refuge in the town's Catholic church. Though the Tutsis padlocked themselves inside the church's iron doors, the Hutu militia forced themselves inside. In this house of God, more than 10,000 people were slaughtered with rifles, machetes, sledgehammers, and grenades. The killing took two days.

The bodies of most victims—along with those of 35,000 others who were murdered in the area—have since been buried in two mass graves behind the church. Above the main entrance, a banner reads in Kinyarwanda: "If you had known me, and you had really known yourself, you would not have killed me."

The building is filled with the victims' clothing and the metallic scent of blood. Each pew is piled high with tattered, red-soaked fabric, while other pieces dangle from clotheslines strung across the room. The white altar cloth is stained with blood. The ceiling is scarred from bullets. A baptismal font has been a witness to more death than life.

The church basement has been converted into a catacomb, lined with racks of bones. Several shelves hold skulls. There are more shelves for femurs and another with arms.

In the room where the children hid, one brick wall is stained with blood. This is where the genocidaires tossed the tiny bodies against the wall. They didn't even bother with machetes.

Whenever there's a tragedy, I've noticed people speak in fragments: "I can't even imagine ..." "Such a shame ..." I don't speak here, but I feel fragmented, a Cubist painting of the spirit that has been dissected and reassembled. This place leaves me breathless and hollow, and I have to work to force air into my lungs again. But it's hard. It's hard to share the same air with the last breaths of the dead, breaths that were wrested from them.

It's also hard to reconcile that as I walk the streets of Rwanda, I share the same air with the people who extracted these lives. The thought leaves me dizzy, and I reach for a wall, my fingertips brushing against the blood shed by people I'll never know.

It is strange to feel untethered in a building where I am surrounded by solid things. Bone and stone and brick. The hard, compacted ground beneath my feet. The tin roof overhead. But I realize the things that make us human are so soft and viscous. Blood and fat and flesh. Mind and spirit. Intangible things. Things that never last, no matter how the lives are ended.

Before I leave, I notice an ID card on the floor, part of a display of the victims' personal effects. The card is stained with dried spots of brown blood. When I peek at the name and photo, I see the man had the same birthday as my brother, May 25, 1965. Any of these ghosts could easily be mine. They could belong to any of us.

On the return to Kigali, I wonder what it would feel like to have a mom who died swiftly instead of seeping away over a period of ten years. Is it better to lose someone quickly? Or to have someone taken slowly? Is grief like peeling off a Band-Aid—better to get it over with?

A few years ago, I got into an argument with my best friend from college about our mothers. I don't remember how it started, only that it ended with us trying to one-up the suffering of the other. She insisted that her mom's three-year, ultimately fatal battle with breast cancer was worse than my mom's extended death from Alzheimer's. Of course, I argued Alzheimer's was the cruelest of diseases.

"My mom was in pain," she said.

"My mom doesn't know she's in pain," I retaliated.

"At least you still have a mom around," she said.

"But my mom doesn't know who I am."

"If I still had a mom, even if she didn't know who I was, I would be grateful," she said.

It's not that simple, I thought. "I don't know how to be a daughter to a woman who doesn't know she's a mother," I said.

It was a dumb fight. Of course there's no hierarchy of suffering, no way to measure the ripples that extend from loss. My friend and I both suffered. And we were both so blinded by our own grief that we bickered about which one of us had been hurt more. A fight that has no winner—and who wants to win that one anyway?

The road is nearly empty of vehicles now, but there are people in the fields and along the road. The driver tells me few buses are running because it is Umuganda, a mandatory community service day held on the last Saturday of every month throughout the country. Each neighborhood selects a project, like painting houses, picking up litter, or preparing the fields for crops, and everybody between the ages of eighteen and sixty-five participates.

Umuganda has a long history in Rwanda, but after the genocide it was implemented by the government with the purpose of uniting Hutu and Tutsi neighbors and fostering a sense of community. It is a reconciliation.

Rwanda is, after all, a small country that has no death penalty. When convicted genocidaires are released from prison, as more and more are every year, many of them return to the village or city where they lived prior to the genocide. So the person who slaughtered your family might be your next-door neighbor.

My mother always told me forgiveness was one of the most important life skills a person could cultivate. I don't know if I have that much forgiveness in me.

A FEW DAYS LATER, I AM AT MY HOSTEL IN KIGALI WHEN the power goes out. For a long minute, it feels like someone hit pause on the city. Music halts. The ceiling fan makes one last, slow swish. Everything is still.

I feel my way down the hallways and onto the patio, where others have gathered. I hear the match strike before I see the quivering light of a citronella candle. All of us encircle the flame.

From this perch on a normal night, it's possible to see all the way down the sweeping hillsides of this neighborhood, past the mansions where the ambassadors live, out to where the houses are smaller, the living quarters denser and more modest. But tonight a velvet drape is dropped from the sky. The lights are blotted out, each home erased. It is an even, inky darkness, the great equalizer.

Someone to my left clunks a bottle on the wooden patio table and announces that it is *waragi*, a Ugandan gin distilled from bananas. There are seven of us regulars at the hostel, now crowded around this one rickety table.

We don't know each other well, but the waragi promises that we are about to become friends.

"The power isn't coming on anytime soon," says Shannon, who has lived in Rwanda longer than any of us. "We might as well drink."

The bottle is passed around clockwise, no glasses. When it gets to me, I tip the bottle to my mouth and feel as though I've been punched in the throat. The waragi is harsh and astringent, the taste as bitter as the smell of rubbing alcohol. When I wheeze, Shannon slides a warm bottle of grape Fanta my way as a chaser. Next time around I anticipate the sting, and the drink doesn't burn as much.

Almost two hours later, the power bursts on with the rude force of a party crasher. The lights are intrusive, but they help us see that the liquor is nearly gone.

We walk arm in arm up the street, hail a taxi, and pile into it. My grasp of the area is fair, because I take long, looping morning walks, but we drive through a part of the city I've never seen before. We arrive at a locals' club called Pasadena.

The club is crowded and humid. Condensation slides down the mirrors on the walls. I don't see people as much as a vibrant kaleidoscope of high heels, stretchy minidresses, shiny shirts, and tight pants.

Someone offers me a martini, and what I receive isn't related in any kingdom, class, or phylum to any martini I've ever known, but I sip it anyway. The DJ plays throbbing Nigerian reggae, mashed up with Prince, Shakira, and Chaka Khan, and I dance for hours. The room pulses with energy, the air musky and sweet.

I am still upright and swaying when I begin to fall asleep. My head bobs, and I can't force my eyes to stay open. I have to go. My friends, however, have more stamina. They decide to stay.

Outside, the air is December cool. Goose bumps stipple my arms. It has rained since we entered the club, and the rugged, potholed road glitters with puddles. Thickets of bushes and trees are obscured by a pea soup of fog.

There are no cabs in sight, and I don't trust a motorcycle taxi in these weather conditions. Plus I am disoriented in this part of town, enough to where I can't even point to the direction of the hostel. I don't know how to get home.

Just then a sizable man in a nice suit taps me on the shoulder and offers me a ride in his posh SUV.

"How much?"

"No charge," he says.

The man must feel my skepticism, because he introduces himself as the owner of the club. His face is round, his smile kind.

"You are my customer," he explains. "It's my responsibility to make sure you get home safe."

This is the math of a traveler: Is it safer to risk slick and curvy streets on the back of a moto taxi in severely reduced visibility? Or put myself inside a stranger's car? As I run the calculations in my head, the man opens the door and gestures for me to get inside.

Defying everything my mother ever taught me, I opt for the SUV. It is dark. I buckle the seat belt, and the man locks the doors. I stare out the window as we drive off.

On the road, we make small talk. He asks how I enjoyed the club. I tell him the music was great, and I loved the festive crowd. He's proud. He tells me he named the place in honor of his brother.

We are now in my neighborhood, driving past the embassies, consulates, and ministry offices of Avenue de la Gendarmerie. The streets are a blank slate. It's long past midnight but not quite day.

"Your brother's name was Pasadena?"

No, he says. Of course not.

Years ago, he says, his brother visited California. When he returned to Kigali, he talked at length about the loveliness of Pasadena. The flowers. The kind people. The quick and easy smiles. He said it was the most beautiful place on earth. Violence broke out shortly after the brother's return. The brother was one of the million Rwandans murdered during the genocide.

We reach the metal fence that surrounds the hostel. I tell the man that I live in California, not too far from Pasadena. He pulls to the side of the road, and he puts the vehicle in park.

"And?" He looks at me, eager but anxious. "Is it as wonderful as my brother says?" When I pause, he grips my face in his big, calloused hands. His fingers tremble, and his eyes search mine. "Does the name honor his memory?"

I am sober now.

To me Pasadena is congested highways, chain restaurants, and parking tickets. I've purchased bath bombs from Lush, and I've sampled craft beer at a shiny bar whose name I don't remember. There are flowers, but they've always looked so phony.

I have taken Pasadena for granted; I do not take this man and his experience for granted. I'm here to say what needs to be true, to help fill the empty spaces, and to offer this man what he has already given me—the tiniest quivering light in the darkness. A way home. And so I look the man in the eye.

"It's the most beautiful place on earth."

THE MAN AT THE TOURISM OFFICE IN KIGALI ASKS WHAT day I'd prefer for my gorilla trek, the next item on my list of things to do for Mom. I purposely choose a Sunday, because this already feels like something holy.

The Sunday of my trek is drizzly, and the Virungas are swathed in mist as fine as cotton candy. Parc National des Volcans is sandwiched near the Rwandan border of Uganda and the Democratic Republic of Congo, a majestic landscape carpeted with flowers and lush greenery and a horizon dominated by volcanoes. The hum of birds and insects acts as a choir.

The last remaining mountain gorillas on earth call this place home, so gorilla treks are tightly regulated by the government. There are ten gorilla families available to visit, and just eight people are permitted to visit each family per day. Some families are far, and several hours of grueling hiking are required to reach them. Others are near the base of the mountains and not difficult to locate. The families are tracked daily, so every guide has a pretty good indication of where to go.

I don't mind working for this, so when all the trekkers are sorted into groups, I say I'm up for a hike. My only request is that I'd like to see babies, which the rangers can't promise. However, I'm hopeful. And when I'm separated into my group, the guide's name is Faith.

We are accompanied by armed rangers because, even though the treks are considered to be safe, there is the potential for danger: namely poachers, interaction with wild animals other than gorillas, and the rebel groups that exist along the border of the DRC. This is also the same land where naturalist Dian Fossey, who researched these endangered animals and wrote *Gorillas in the Mist*, was murdered by unknown assailants.

The hike is difficult. I'm given my own machete, and we slog through knee-high mud and thick tangles of stinging nettles. My clothes aren't thick, and I am tagged, poked, snagged by thorns, even as I try to slice my way through branches and vines. When the climb gets particularly steep, I use the machete to carve steps into the mud. And when the mountain grows too steep for that, I climb on all fours, gorilla-style, clinging to bamboo stalks to keep myself from sliding away. When I stand again, my boots are heavy and feel as though they've been dipped in molasses.

None of that matters when we encounter the gorilla. He's just there, sitting on his haunches in a little clearing, surrounded by bushes. He's close enough that I can hear him breathe and smell the musk of his fur.

Then there are gorillas everywhere, eating, playing, climbing. Some of them frolic and run. Others are preoccupied with food. One gorilla snaps a thorny vine, the same kind I had trouble chopping with a machete, and plucks off all the berries.

This is the Umubano family, which means "neighborliness" or "living together," comprised of more than a dozen members. It's an ironic name since this family was initially part of another group, Amahoro. As Charles the silverback grew older, he challenged the more mature silverback in his family, and he eventually left with two females to start his own group.

I'm delighted to see babies, lovable black bundles of fuzz. Just like human infants, these babies don't entirely know how to control their limbs yet, so every movement is equally awkward and hilarious. One baby scratches his head and tips over. Another tries to swing from one tree to another and doesn't make it, crashing into the bushes.

Then I watch mama gorillas nurture their young, with babies on their backs or nestled in the crook of an arm. One of the adult gorillas flattens the foliage into a nest and places her baby there to rest. When the child is good and comfortable, the mama perches nearby where she can keep watch.

I see all this, and even as I marvel at the gorillas, I also think, *Nope. Not me.* I recall the children I met in Argentina, how much I wanted to protect them, but here I waver. I don't know if I'm capable of caring for a child this way; I don't know if I have the capacity for selflessness. I'm the machete wielder, not the nurturer. I am hard where I should be tender.

My only instinct is the one that tells me to stay calm as Charles the silverback swaggers past me. He places one enormous hand, as large as a baseball mitt, on my shoulder. Faith whispers, "Don't move," and Charles continues moving forward. Then he pauses at the edge of a clearing that looks over the mountain below and surveys the landscape.

Neatly side by side, the gorilla and I gaze past the skinny trees, the scruffy bushes, the thorny, creeping vines, down the ragged green hills. Wispy clouds shift past us. My forearms are streaked in mud, scrapes, and dried blood, but my muscles are relaxed; the discomfort I experienced getting here has dissipated. There is no sound but my own heartbeat. I hesitate to blink, too afraid of breaking the stillness and the sanctity of this moment.

Do I even need to tell you I feel alive?

It's my final day in Rwanda. My backpack is crammed all the way to the top with gifts for my family—necklaces made with paper beads, hand-sewn dolls, a small chess set that looked so pretty in the shadows of the market but is actually just a square of floor tile and some lumps of plastic.

There's only one thing left to do: teach my final class. I've recently introduced them to the game of bingo—we play using boards that I've made with English vocabulary words, and the students cover the squares with rusty bottle caps.

When class ends, a few students offer to take me out. We board a bus to a nearby neighborhood, then walk down a dirt lane to a small restaurant.

The building is slender, barely large enough to hold the kitchen's few burners. All the tables are located outside, on a dirt patio surrounded by wooden fences and tarps with beer advertisements. I am the only non-Rwandan. The other customers stare.

At the table, one student pulls a pack of Uno cards from her pocket and asks if I can show them how to play.

I shuffle the cards and deal seven to each woman, just as a waitress arrives. Liberé orders several large beers and plates of French fries, *mizuzu* (fried plantains), and goat brochettes (skewers) for the table. We play an open hand.

All the vocabulary words my class worked so hard to learn seem to come together in this game: color words, directions, numbers. I have to explain the concept of a "wild" card, and there's a little bit of confusion over "skip"—which my students only know as the physical movement of hopping. Otherwise, they've got it.

Our food arrives, and the fries sizzle and pop with oil. We continue playing Uno, laughing and discarding onto the plastic table, the cards now greasy with thumbprints. It's early, but the sky is already a steely gray.

We draw a small crowd with our game. The server looks over our shoulders and makes suggestions for what to discard. A couple of other people pull up chairs and watch, laughing whenever one of us shatters the night with a scream of "UNO!"

We've played maybe six or seven rounds when the rain begins. It's only a light drizzle at first, just enough to make the table get slick, the dirt smell mossy, my curly red hair go boing. By the time Francoise stacks the Uno cards together and shoves them inside her pocket, we're sitting in a full-fledged storm.

The restaurant is already crammed with people—there's no way we can squeeze inside. Claudette tugs my hand and pulls me beneath a small blue awning near the building. Liberé and Francoise pile around me.

The harder the rain falls, the more physically uncomfortable I become. I need to use the restroom in the worst way.

"Toilet is there," Liberé says, and she points to a small shelter made from scraps of metal hammered together. It has no roof. At first I think she's joking, but the other students also cast their eyes downward and shake their heads.

The sky shows no sign of clearing, and there are no other buildings nearby. And using the toilet has become the most important thing in the world.

Liberé pushes her way inside the restaurant and emerges with three different umbrellas. She hands one to Claudette and one to Francoise and keeps one for herself. She jerks her head toward the toilet. "We go," she says.

These women encircle me, forming a wall with their bodies, and we move across the muddy lot as one creature. The mud squishes between my feet and my flip-flops, and I almost slip. My students squeeze me so tight, they never let me fall.

At the metal building, I use the small flashlight from my purse to peer inside. One side is completely exposed where there should have been a door. The ground is a slurry of muck. I still want to use the toilet, but it looks treacherous, and I don't know if I can hold myself upright.

Claudette leans over the top of the structure and holds her umbrella there to form a roof. Francoise blocks part of the open door space with her body, allowing me privacy, even though there's nobody around. Liberé faces me and extends her hand.

"Hold me," she says.

I am so exposed—my khaki pants pulled down my thighs, my underwear down, perched on the edge of a sludgy slope, raindrops sliding down the side of my face. I think about my girlfriends in California, how we scurry to the bathroom in groups to gossip and touch up our makeup. We preen in front of shiny mirrors and share secrets. It's not so different, these fleeting moments of intimacy.

I hold my hand out to grasp Liberé's, and she ropes her fingers tightly through mine.

   If these women want to hurt me, this is the perfect opportunity. They could abandon me at this restaurant, far from the places I know. They could do anything—let me get soaked, mock me, taunt me. Instead Liberé gives my hand a squeeze. She's got me.

Heaven and Earth Meet Halfway

⊰⊱

IT TAKES ONE FULL DAY OF TRAVEL BY BUS, PLANE, AND
taxi to arrive at my next destination: a hostel near Tahrir Square, the major
public space in downtown Cairo.

The hostel is located five stories up in a gritty building. Inside, the
ground level looks like rubble, with broken stone, brick, and rubbish piled
against the walls, which are decorated with spurts of graffiti. It looks like the
place has been hit by artillery. The stairs are blocked by tape, so I'm forced
to use the elevator, which looks to be about 150 years old. It's a cage of black
wrought iron, a rickety old thing that screeches as it moves. I close my eyes as
I am slowly and loudly lifted to the proper floor.

The door of the hostel looks like a prop from a film noir, something
more suited to a hard-boiled detective's office. It's a wooden half-light door
with pebbled glass, but where it might say "Sam Spade" in gold letters, there
is a sign with Arabic words. Underneath that, in black marker, is scrawled
"HOTLE."

Inside the door is a tall wooden desk, like that of a bank teller, manned by a plump guy in a brown robe. When I give my name, the man raises an eyebrow. My reservation is for two, but I'm clearly alone.

"My husband will be joining me later," I say, and I thrill at the sound of those words. It's been six long months since I've seen Jason, and I can't remember the last time I used the phrase "my husband" to describe him. At this point, we've spent more of our marriage apart than together.

With some financial assistance from my family, Jason gathered enough money to visit me for Christmas, and we agreed upon Cairo for our rendezvous. As a teacher, he has almost two weeks off for the winter holidays. Minus flying time and a couple days for jet lag, we have just over one week together, and I'm ecstatic.

I reserved a room with a queen-sized bed, but when I unlock the door I see two twin beds.

I return to the front desk. "There must be a mistake," I say, and the man in the robe follows me to the room.

"No, no mistake," he says. "Two beds make queen."

It's not the same, I explain. "I haven't seen my husband in many months."

"Eh, I understand," the man laughs lasciviously, then gives me a firm slap on the back. "You want . . . ," he pauses, then makes a circle with the fingers of his left hand, which he penetrates with the index finger of his other hand. "Poke poke, yes?"

I roll my eyes, but my face burns red.

"No problem," the man says, gesturing to the beds. "Push together."

The man gums his cigarette while he pushes the two twin beds together, and ashes sprinkle down upon the thin maroon bedspreads. This situation dashes my hopes for a romantic reunion—cuddling in a big, luxurious bed, falling asleep with our limbs tangled together, waking in each other's arms. Instead, Jason and I will be tucked in to separate spaces with separate sheets, a definitive line cutting our bed right down the middle. But it beats sleeping on the airport floor, like we did in Peru.

Once the man leaves, I have some time to look around. The walls of the room have been painted to resemble the inside of a pyramid. From the window, I have a good view of the city, which already looks far more chaotic than when I arrived. What was once four lanes of traffic has now become seven, all trying to merge together. The streets shoot off each other at bizarre angles, and they are crowded with street carts, people, cars, donkeys, and buses. It's almost 7 p.m., and it seems like everyone in Cairo has someplace to be.

That includes me. I didn't realize I was hungry until I look down and see a line of people purchasing freshly fried falafel from a street vendor. I rush to join them—holding my breath as the creaky elevator lowers me back to earth.

When I take a deep breath outside, the air is clogged and dirty and smells of burning tires. It is loud and messy, but also lively and exciting. I can't squelch the feeling that something big is going to happen here.

IT IS JUST AFTER 4 A.M. WHEN I WAKE.

The sheet has been pulled away from my body, and a man skims his fingertips over me. It's a light touch, like a butterfly wing or a feather, but the strangeness of it makes me stiffen.

"I've missed you," Jason says; then he bends over to give me a kiss.

I don't know how to react. It's been six months since my lips have kissed someone back. Six months since I've savored the scent of a man's neck. Six months since I've been held. Jason eases himself into the twin bed next to mine.

"I'm sorry about the bed," I say. I feel nervous and shy, like we've just met. "I tried to …"

"Shhh," Jason says. "I'm just happy to see you."

He tugs on a lock of my hair and curls it around his finger. He's just looking at me. I stare back, like I'm trying to interpret the hidden meaning of an abstract painting.

"Hi." I can't stop saying hi. I once heard that goldfish only have two-second memories, so they just swim around in their fishbowl, reintroducing themselves over and over again. I feel like that now.

The moonlight illuminates his smile, and my insides go warm.

The line the beds make between us is definitive, but the distance is not insurmountable.

IT TAKES A FEW DAYS FOR MY BODY TO REGAIN THE MUSCLE memory of Jason, but when I do, it's like we haven't spent any time apart.

We make a small loop around the country, starting with Cairo, where we wander the long, rambling hallways of the Egyptian Museum. There are few information cards posted with the exhibitions; sometimes there's just a yellowed index card with a typewritten name or date. Some of the pieces have no display at all. We lose ourselves among tables of unidentified mummies, stone panels of hieroglyphs on the floor, broken statues shoved in the corner. Wooden cargo boxes are stacked high nearby. It makes me feel like I'm an Egyptologist in the 1920s, sifting through these artifacts for the first time. Clouds of dust make me sneeze.

I run my finger along a stone carving made by someone thousands of years ago, and I recall the first time I learned that Egypt was a real place: when I was a child in church.

My mom has always been a devout Lutheran, and she carried a fancy study Bible, the kind with a pebbled leather cover, embossed gold words, and thumb indexes for each chapter. Her Bible also contained a maps insert with a 30,000-foot aerial view of biblical lands, the terrain filled with arrows depicting possible routes where Moses traveled and Jesus walked, annotated with Bible verses.

Those were stories, though, and I'd heard plenty of stories. A talking snake. A burning bush. People raised from the dead.

But the photographs in the insert were real. That included an image of the pyramids of Giza—a backdrop of barren, gold desert; colossal, perfectly symmetrical pyramids rising toward the pale sky; camels in the foreground, small dots in comparison to the monuments. I had many questions.

"They're the Great Pyramids, and they're a wonder of the world," my mom explained. "I'll take you there someday."

When Jason and I spend a day in Giza, I know I'm doing something my mother wanted to do—and wanted to do with me.

Giza, however, unsettles me. The pyramids themselves are grand, arranged on a carpet of the finest sand. They were built to withstand time, and that's what they've done, though the structures look incongruous surrounded by urban development and modern litter.

It strikes me as strange to honor my mother by walking through enormous tombs. That's why the pyramids were created, after all. The pharaohs expected to become gods in the afterlife, and they erected massive tombs that contained everything they needed to rule. And here I am, paying to walk around in their necropolis.

What I can appreciate is the shape of the pyramid itself, supposed to represent the physical body leaving earth and ascending toward the sun. I don't even know if I believe in an afterlife, but I like the continuity that exists within that idea, the concept that the spirit will be engaged in something mightier than this realm.

When I first moved to California, I got a life coach. She was a gray-haired grandmotherly type, as likely to send me off with a linty butterscotch candy from her pocket as a piece of quartz and a bundle of sage. She believed life was as pliable as Play-Doh, and it was a person's responsibility to sculpt his or her life into what he or she wanted. During our sessions, I told her how my mom's suffering was making me suffer, how badly I wanted her pain to end.

"It's time," the coach said. "It's time for your mom to go, but she doesn't realize it yet. Her body is lingering on this plane because she has no clear path out. You have to be the one to tell her. She needs your permission to leave. Tell her it's okay to go."

She insisted that these words needed to be whispered in my mom's ear, and that they would inspire her spirit to move forward to the next phase.

"Only when this pain ends will you be your most authentic self," the life coach said.

It would be months before I was back in Ohio, and my authentic self couldn't wait that long. I called my sister and told her exactly what the life coach said. The idea was that these words would slice through the disease and connect with Mom's spirit. I imagined her like a cicada, shedding this unnecessary shell and taking flight. My sister agreed that she would say the words to our mom the next time she was at the nursing home.

"It's time to go," my sister told Mom. "It's okay. We'll be fine. You can go."

My mom didn't answer. That was four years ago, and only the life coach has departed my realm, because I fired her.

Inside the pyramids, Jason and I scramble through narrow corridors and airless rooms. It is hot. So cramped. To see the Sphinx, the famed monument with the head of a pharaoh on the body of a lion, we walk past lines of vendors shoving postcards and souvenirs in our faces. We are offered twenty-seven camel rides. Policemen speak to us in whispers—they can take us into the closed pyramids for a special price. Just five dollars to climb all over these priceless structures. For ten dollars, they will take our picture.

Jason is overwhelmed by the aggressiveness, the way the touts look at us and see money, how people follow us and beg. I try to make it easier on him, and when I see vendors approach, I give them a firm "No." Sometimes it works.

I buy our bus tickets, haggle at the market, hail taxis, navigate the Metro. I locate food, figure out directions, quickly calculate currency conversions in my head.

Jason is amazed. "Where did you learn to do this?" he says. "I've never seen you so in control."

I shrug, but I'm secretly proud. These six months have made me more confident and assertive. If my mom were still aware of the world around her, and if she passed me on the street, what would she think?

Jason and I take the night train to Luxor in a private compartment with bunk beds. When we wake in the morning, we notice a small bullet hole in our window. The cracks that radiate from it make a beautiful pattern, an intricate spiderweb.

"Do you think we're in danger?" Jason asks. He's read too many travel books with warnings about attacks on American tourists.

I'm not concerned. If there was any danger, we've long ago passed it in the night. "Just pretend this is an Agatha Christie novel," I say.

Over the course of a few days, we sightsee our way down the Nile— Luxor, Esna, Edfu, Aswan, Abu Simbel. Finally, on Christmas, we catch a short flight to Sharm el-Sheikh, then take a taxi to Dahab, a sleepy village on the Red Sea.

It is only once we reach Dahab that I truly relax into Jason again, redis- covering the part of my identity that is his partner, not just a tour guide. We hold hands the way we used to, and once again it feels comfortable to have someone by my side. It's taken a few days, but we are no longer strangers.

Dahab is a hippie town, located on a small crescent of the Sinai Pen- insula, where the desert mountains run out of momentum and give way to sand. The blue water is lit up with teal swaths of coral reef, and the weather is warm almost all year long.

"I'm already happy here," Jason says.

"Me too." I give his hand a squeeze.

Though some are dressed modestly, most are not. Many men are in shorts and T-shirts, while the women wear swimsuits, sarongs, or gauzy sun- dresses. This is the first place in Egypt where I feel comfortable removing the head scarf I've worn since Cairo.

Signs on the beach prohibit camels and horses, though I see both on the boardwalk nearby. Ladies in brightly colored bikinis tan themselves on sun-bleached blankets and cushions. Groups of scuba divers, about eight to twelve in each pack, waddle from dive shops into the sea and disappear into its depths. A few strings of tinsel are the only visual nods to the holiday.

Christmas was always a big deal for my mom, who threw herself into the preparations with the enthusiasm and dedication of a military commander. I, however, had to be coerced to help. Arranging the branches on the artificial tree made me itchy, the ornaments were ugly and old, the treetop angel was losing her hair. And the bane of my childhood existence? Strands of silver icicles that my mom wanted placed on the tree, one by one.

Then we decorated the house. There were ribbons and candles, na- tivity scenes and Advent calendars, holly-shaped candy dishes and special tablecloths trimmed in red and green. The centerpiece involved enormous pinecones that my mom collected and adorned with glitter. She sprayed the windowpanes with fake snow. She thought it was fun; I thought it was tacky.

She was happiest on Christmas Eve, and my most vivid holiday memories live in that space, contained in a snow globe of time. Every year we attended church together, the late service, just her and me. Each congregant was given a small, unlit candle, about the size of a dry-erase marker, which we held on to throughout the entire service in a darkened sanctuary. Then during the final hymn, "Silent Night," the pastor plucked a candle from the altar and used it to light the candle of someone in the front row. That person used his or her candle to light another, and so on, until the entire church pulsed with flickering light.

I can shake that snow globe and see that moment fall into place again and again: My mom bending toward me, soft cheeks and red lips radiant and illuminated, gently tipping her candle to avoid spilling wax. I hold my breath. Her fire ignites mine. She tells me to wait until my flame is strong before I pass it on.

In Dahab, Jason and I settle into a small café with a wooden patio overlooking the water, where we prop ourselves up on fat pillows. The waiter welcomes us with a hearty "Merry Christmas!" followed up with something that sounds like a dyslexic Santa, "Oh oh oh!" He brings us pita bread, hummus, falafel, slices of cucumber, and squat mugs of coffee. A stray cat, orange and scrawny, settles at my feet. I sneak him pieces of pita bread, and he purrs so forcefully that my legs vibrate.

In the afternoon, Jason and I visit an internet café to call our families over Skype. Today my dad is at my sister's house, where her husband sets up the computer so the whole family can see me. My college-aged nephews stand in the background, and my brother-in-law offers a quick wave. My sister and I catch up; she's jealous of my Egyptian tan. Finally, my dad pulls an armchair up to the computer.

My dad doesn't know how to operate the camera on his computer, so even though I've talked to him over the phone, this is the first time I've seen his face in months. His eyes are hooded, and his cheeks are sunken and drawn. I am alarmed.

He says he's okay, but his flat, dull tone belies his own words. He reports that my mom is fine and that she had a nice holiday in the nursing home. It's not long before he excuses himself and I'm left staring at a blank, black screen.

That night, before I fall asleep, my side feels pinched, and my breath is strained. I can't shake the nagging feeling something isn't right.

I HAVE ONLY TWO HOURS OF SLEEP BEFORE JASON SHAKES me awake to board an unmarked van. We barrel through the desert in this chilly vehicle full of strangers, until it stops at the base of a mountain. Our trek to the top of Mount Sinai begins at 1 a.m., led by a Bedouin guide.

There are two routes to the summit. We take the camel path, a wide trail that snakes its way to the summit at a more gentle, gradual pace than the alternative, the steep 3,750 Steps of Penitence.

We walk for hours through the inky blackness of night, and it feels good. Hiking is where Jason and I hit our most comfortable stride, our feet moving across the ground one step at a time, slowly making our way forward. When his foot slides on loose rock, my arm instinctively juts out to steady him. When my lungs feel weak, he rests with me.

Together we pass Bedouin men, sprawled out on woven rugs, selling lanterns. A chain of camels follows behind us, some of them wearing brass bells that cut through the desert silence. We stop for several minutes in a small shelter, a cave carved like a deep trough into the gray mountain, where an old woman sells hot tea. It is cold, and the woman wraps us in donkey blankets as we thaw our fingers around the hot mugs.

The final push to the summit consists of 700 stone steps. There are many other hikers and pilgrims around us now. The old and weak dismount camels and then take the stairs slowly, lingering over each one. The young lean against boulders. Other than wheezy gasps for air, everyone is silent.

Jason and I make it to the top and find a flat place to sit. It has taken more than three hours to climb about three miles up this mountain—the second highest in Egypt—with an elevation gain of approximately 2,500 feet. The air is frigid, and we wrap our arms around each other. The sky is navy, and my breath forms little clouds.

When I was a little girl and attended church with my mom, I wrote letters to God during the service on prayer-request slips. But I didn't hand these prayers over with the offering plate, like everyone else did. To me, nature felt like a more direct line to God. So I tucked my letters away and only handed them over later, when I was in my backyard or at the creek that gurgled through our neighborhood. I hid my prayers under stones; I tucked them into trees. I asked God to find my letters and answer me.

Now I'm at the peak of Sinai, the place where Moses is said to have received the tablets containing the Ten Commandments. If there is any place in the world where my words will reach God, this is it. I fold my hands together, and I wait.

This peak is where I silently pray—I ask for love and compassion, I ask for my family's good health, I ask for my mom to be at peace. And then I express my gratitude: For this sacred night on a mountain with the man I love. For the people I've met along my journey and the radical acts of kindness I've received. For this earth that makes a full rotation every day and somehow always finds the sun again.

Dawn comes like a slash in the sky, as if a knife sliced right through a yard of dark fabric. As the rip of sky widens, revealing pastel orange, pink, and finally yellow, a deep hum begins, a sound both warm and resonant.

There is a small stone mosque and a Greek Orthodox church near the flat rock where Jason and I sit. The Muslim call to prayer and the Christian hymns begin simultaneously, creating a chorus of praise in an otherworldly harmony. It is an appropriate soundtrack to the morning, as the sun paints the desolate desert landscape below a dramatic pink.

I wouldn't call myself religious, but I do say I'm spiritual, and watching the dark earth unfolding into a rich, vibrant world is something as close to transcendent as I've ever witnessed. No wonder Moses and God used this as their meeting point. This place feels like a bridge across time, a span between two worlds.

Jason and I continue to hold each other. My head rests against his chest, and he strokes my hair. I don't know why I begin to cry.

A part of me must already know that when I travel back down the mountain, I will have left this sacred place perched at the edge of the sky—this pause between heaven and earth—to face cold reality. By the time I reach the lower desert again, I will have just two more days with my husband, my father will have sent terrible news, and nothing will ever be the same again.

DEATH

Bedenke dass du sterben musst. (Remember that you have to die.)

—German memento mori

Eat the Camel

Egyptian traffic is loud, fast-moving, and nonstop, separating me from the market where I can get food. I whip my head around, searching for a crosswalk, a traffic light, a traffic cop, even a traffic *sign*. Anything that will help me move from one side of the street to the other. But I'm staring down vehicular anarchy in a swollen city, where 22 million people stretch the limits of streets built for 4 million.

Somehow other people manage to navigate this mess. Men wearing airy galabeyas, women in hijabs, students sporting smart gray suits, and even children brave the road. They find a kind of harmony in the chaos, establishing eye contact with the drivers, walking at a steady pace—moving *shway shway*, slowly slowly, across one lane at a time—until they are absorbed into the traffic flow.

Just when I'm about to give up, I meet Rami.

"There is trick," he says, standing along my right elbow. He is shaped like a stout light bulb, with a shiny bald head and wide smile.

"Really?"

He giggles. "Close your eyes and pray to Allah."

With that, he takes my arm and pulls me into the current.

Afterward, we sit together at a street café, sipping mint tea in mugs the size of shot glasses and smoking apple-flavored tobacco in a hookah. Rami asks about my family, but I can't summon the words to explain my story.

I just tell him that I'm backpacking.

When Rami invites me to stay at his family's house in Giza, I say yes. I'm overwhelmed by his generosity—opening his door for a stranger on the street—but more than that, in a world that is infinite and strange and beautiful, I'm still searching for some semblance of home. Here is someone willing to embrace me as one of his own, and I'm touched.

I also don't have anywhere else to go. New Year's Eve is approaching, the hostels are booked, and my budget is too meager for the city's pricier options. Just that morning a hostel owner said he was going to kick me out to make room for someone with a reservation. I was only in Cairo to see Jason off, and without him the city has a film of sadness.

After Rami and I pick up my backpack, we are met by Rami's uncle, Sabar, a wiry thirtysomething. He arrives in a beat-up sedan and barely stops moving long enough to let us climb inside.

In a particularly congested part of the city, Sabar rolls down the window with a hand crank and plops a fake, magnetic police light on the roof. He presses a couple of buttons, launching an assault of sirens and flashing lights.

"Makes cars go away!" Sabar laughs.

With traffic, the drive from Cairo to Giza is fifty minutes. We get there in ten. Underneath a bridge, Sabar pulls over, and Rami and I continue navigating the maze to his house. I have been traveling alone for six months, so long gone into the world that I am no longer actively afraid of it; my body holds the same low simmer of fear here as it does at home, the ever-present anxiety of being a woman who exists. So I am not scared to go with Rami. But I am aware, always aware.

There is a lurching public bus, which takes us just a few blocks. Then we hop into a sputtering rickshaw and weave through traffic—this time scooters and donkey carts—down shadowed alleyways, behind rows of identical concrete buildings. Finally, Rami and I walk a little over a mile on roads too narrow for the rickshaw to negotiate.

The paths are made of compacted dirt, raised slightly above chunky sewage and stagnant water. Garbage clogs the canals, and dead animal carcasses rot on the piles of trash. Rami and I press on through clouds of bloated flies, past unmarked stores and cafés, through the smoke of burning rubber. I never see any street signs.

"Is okay?" Rami says.

"Is fine, is fine," I say, keeping my doubts to myself. I have no cell service. I doubt there's an internet connection for my laptop. Nobody knows where I am. I don't even know.

From the outside, Rami's three-story house looks abandoned. Stalks of rebar jut out from the top. Windows are broken. The front door is raised a couple of feet from the ground, but there are no steps to get there. I'm tall, and it requires a mighty stretch and Rami's assistance to get in the door. We kick off our shoes and make two neat piles at the foot of the staircase.

The family lives on the second level. The concrete floor of the living room is draped with a rug so thin, it looks like a whisper. There is little furniture.

Rami's mother has been expecting us. She greets me with two sheets of newspaper rolled into a cone. Inside are hot, fried falafel the size of flattened ice cream scoops, wrapped in warm pita bread. Oil soaks through the paper and makes my hands hot and greasy. The crust of each falafel is slightly burnt, which heightens the texture of the soft, warm middle. Flecks of parsley are so fresh they taste like the color green.

"Best chef in Egypt!" Rami beams, and I agree. It is the best I've ever had, and I've eaten a lot of falafel.

When I'm finished, Rami rolls the oily newspapers from our meal into a ball, along with some food waste, wilted vegetables, and bones. We carry it to the roof, where the goats live, and feed our scraps to the animals. Whatever the goats can't eat—like an empty potato chip bag—is tossed off the roof, where it joins the other trash blowing through the streets.

It is dusk, and the street below is illuminated with few lights. A boy walks by with a burlap sack that squirms and whines. Puppies.

"Where is he taking them?" I ask. I feel my voice rise with notes of panic.

"They will drown," Rami says. "But do not worry. Better to be dead than live in Giza."

As much as I don't want the puppies to die, in the ten years my mom has spent dying, I've grown to understand that ending life can be more merciful than letting it continue. Many times I wondered why my mom continued to survive, why her body pressed on without her in it, why we couldn't let this vibrant, beautiful woman go with dignity instead of acting as bystanders to her decline. I've learned our culture is not necessarily one of compassion. We champion those who suffer, even while we don't want to suffer ourselves.

It's been one day since my mom was moved into hospice care, a fact I learned when Jason and I returned from our Mount Sinai trek. My dad emailed to say my mom wouldn't live much longer.

He wrote:

Margaret, I didn't want to tell you this on Christmas, so I waited a couple of days. Mom has taken a turn for the worse. About a week ago she started having trouble swallowing. We tried a medicine to encourage her appetite, but all it did was cause her to sleep. It was difficult to wake her up again, so we have stopped the medicine. I have no idea when the rest of her vital organs will stop working. Now you know. Love, Dad.

We decided a long time ago that we wouldn't put my mom on a feeding tube, so it is only a matter of time before she succumbs to starvation.

Now my mom's impending death feels like the traffic in Cairo. Chaotic. Daunting. I am unable to weave my way through the lanes, so far from finding footing on the other side. I ask my dad if I should come home, and he says I shouldn't bother. She won't know I'm there. She doesn't know anything at all.

Rami abruptly leaves to meet friends, and his sister, Raina, is on the phone with her boyfriend. That leaves me with the matriarch, her three sisters, and an in-law, and none of them speak English. Rami's mother turns on the TV and adjusts the rabbit-ear antennas until a show appears. Based on the dramatic expressions and swelling music, I assume this is an Arabic soap opera.

I watch the TV show this way, five women forming almost a complete circle around me, and still I feel alone. What I wouldn't give to watch *The Young and the Restless* or *Guiding Light* with my mom again. I choke back a sob. One woman shoots me a stern look, raises a finger to her lips, and spits as she shushes. They scoot away from me, and there's a hollow, lonely space where these women used to be.

WE SLEEP THAT NIGHT ON THE LIVING ROOM FLOOR, ALL of us jumbled together like a cluttered drawer of cutlery: Rami, his mother, her sisters, the daughters, some friends of the family, and the one in-law. We wrap itchy wool blankets around our bodies, burrito style. I smash one of my sweaters into a ball, and that serves as my pillow. Raina, next to me, curls under a tented blanket to talk on the phone with her boyfriend.

Mosquitoes hum near my ears, and bigger swarms swish the air around my head. I tighten the blanket around my face. Mosquitoes land on my cheeks. I pull the blanket tighter again, until only my mouth and nostrils are bare, and I inhale insects. They fly into my mouth and sting my lips. I pull the blanket over my head until I can barely breathe.

In the morning, my skin is swollen. My face, arms, and legs are covered with bites. I point to the hot, pink welts that line my limbs. The family shrugs. The mosquitoes did not touch them. Raina jokes, "Is because you are so sweet."

I don't have any lotions or creams to offer relief, and I don't know where to buy any. The only medicine in my backpack is a small vial of *sangre de grado*, dragon's blood, that I received from a shaman in the Amazon rainforest six months earlier. The dragon's blood is the dark, red resin of a tree, said to be therapeutic for skin ailments and infection.

That morning, while my mother is in Ohio taking some of her last, ragged breaths on earth, I smear dragon's blood on my body, staining my skin a menstrual red-brown. There are twenty-seven spots on my face, including three on my lips, seventeen on my left arm, twelve on my right. My legs are even worse, so gnawed that I lose count of the welts. Later I catch sight of my reflection in a decorative urn. I look bloody and beaten. I don't even recognize myself.

Raina looks at me with dismay. She is a devout Muslim teen who dresses modestly in turtlenecks and floor-length skirts. But she is also stylish, donning a lacy tank top over her turtleneck, pulling on bright tights underneath her skirt, draping a decorative scarf over her plain, black hijab. And because Raina thinks everything is better with a little sparkle, she drapes layers of necklaces around her neck and slips stacks of glittery bracelets over her wrists. It looks like she purchases rhinestones in bulk.

Finally Raina says, "My mother is mad at you."

"Why? What have I done?"

"You blame us for bites on your skin," she says. "You think we are dirty. You hate staying with us."

"No, I don't blame you, and I don't think you are dirty," I say. "These bites hurt very much. I am in pain."

"You hate us."

"No, I don't," I insist. "I'm just sad."

Raina suggests a shower to feel better, and those are magic words. It has been months since I've had the kind of shower I was accustomed to in the United States. Backpacking around Africa, I took a lot of bucket baths, which are exactly what they sound like—standing over a drain or on a dirt floor with a bucket of water, running a bar of soap over my skin, using a small cup to dump the water all over my body.

While eco-friendly and efficient, bucket baths are not enjoyable. Not the way I enjoy showers at home. I imagine the slap of hot water on my sore skin. Lathering my hair with shampoo. Letting the water stream over my head and face and shoulders, washing all the dirt and hurt away.

Raina tells me to be patient. The shower will be ready soon. The rest of the family has disappeared, Raina leaves the room, and I wait alone. After about an hour, Raina leads me by the hand into the bathroom.

The bathroom has a toilet, though it can only be flushed by pouring a bucket of water into the tank. There is also a bathtub, though it is filled with plastic chairs, boxes, and assorted dishes.

"Where is the shower?" I ask.

"Stand here," Raina says, positioning me near the toilet. The floor is tile, slanted toward a single drain. Raina leaves the room and returns carrying a fat metal pot of water. She places the pot on the floor, shuts the door, and instructs me to remove my clothes.

"But shower . . . ?" I say.

"Here is shower."

She balances on top of the toilet seat, holding a measuring cup with a long handle. One cup at a time, water is poured on my head. Each tiny cascade is near boiling, hot enough to make my flesh sting. All the while, Raina sings in Arabic. The tune is sweet and mournful.

"My mother is dying," I say.

"Everybody dies," Raina says; then she continues to sing.

"No, I mean my mother is dying. Right now," I say. "She is in a hospital in Ohio. She might already be dead."

"Everybody dies," Raina says again. "Life is to suffer."

"I thought I already lost her," I continue. "But I was wrong."

Raina dribbles shampoo on my head and combs her fingers through the ropes of my curly hair. Then, with a firm hand, she runs a bar of heavily perfumed soap over my body and rubs my skin until it lathers. When she rinses me, I am pink. I have never felt so naked.

After the shower, I towel off and dress. Raina takes me by the hand and leads me to her room, where I sit on a cardboard box. She combs the tangles of my hair and pulls it back into a taut, low-slung ponytail, then covers my head with a gray hijab. On top of that, she winds a purple silky scarf and secures the ends with a rhinestone brooch.

"Oh my, very nice," she says, nodding in approval.

She applies concealer to the mosquito bites on my face and slathers on several layers of foundation meant for olive complexions, a stark contrast to my pale skin. The rest of the makeover looks like the kind of makeup I applied at my mother's vanity as a small girl. Penciled eyebrows. Streaks of magenta blush. Layers of shiny blue eye shadow that rain sparkly dust onto my cheeks. Lips fat and pink. I am Raina's life-sized American Girl doll.

"Now you look so pretty," she says. "Ah yes. Very good."

For the final touch, she decorates me with costume jewelry. Purple-studded bracelets. Necklaces of green plastic beads, cut to look like diamonds. A tarnished metal ring with a stone like a Ping-Pong ball.

Raina steps back and appraises her work. "I cannot take you outside," she decides. "All the mens will be looking."

By now, the rest of the family has returned to the house. I hear a symphony of sounds from the kitchen, the next room over, where the mother is working with the other women. The thud of a knife against wood. A rattle from a heavy, boiling pot. The scrape of pestle against mortar. A strange man arrives and hands paper-wrapped packages to the mother, who disappears into the kitchen once again.

When it is time to eat, there is no table. Instead Raina shows me how to spread a layer of newspapers on the floor. The entire family gathers and squats around the paper. The mother—one plump, bare foot bent under her body, the other sticking straight out, resting against a platter of salad—nods with approval at my makeover.

They fill my plate until it is heavy, heaped with white rice, fava beans, chopped cucumber salad, and the bitter, soupy greens of *mulukhiyah*. In the center of it all is a thick ball of grilled meat, bigger than my hand, slick with hot, hissing juice. I realize I never told them I am a vegetarian.

I politely nibble around the meat. "Oh, I am not so hungry. I cannot eat all this," I say, and I rub my belly with one hand. I offer it to Rami. "Maybe you would like my meat?"

But this is New Year's Eve. Even though this Bedouin family doesn't celebrate the holiday, they know it is a special day for my culture, and I am their guest.

"Very special for you," Rami says.

He says the family slaughtered their uncle's camel and saved the liver for me. It's a delicacy.

"Eat, eat," the mother urges.

This family offers me sustenance on a platter, even as the woman who nourished me lies starving. At this moment it is my decision to devour the food or to deny it, but I realize my mom has no choice.

All eyes look to me with anticipation. I take a bite. I close my eyes. I chew. The camel tastes like a punch in the face. Dark and heavy, metal and blood. It is both primal and complex. Something like life itself.

Brittle Stars

⸻⸙⸻

AFTER I LEAVE RAMI'S HOUSE, I MAKE MY WAY BACK TO Dahab. My intention is to rent a place for a little while, hunker down, let my broken spirit and tired body heal. Maybe I'll do some writing.

I am in desperate need of a place to call home when I stumble across a temporary private room at a little yoga camp, which is where I become friends with Katie. I'm there when I receive an email from my dad that shocks me. My grandmother in Germany—my mom's mom, and the only grandparent I've ever known—has passed away.

My dad's messages are like him, rigid and no-nonsense, and he doesn't offer any details about her death. Even so, it sends me reeling, so the people at the yoga camp envelop me with kindness and tenderly guide me through my loss. Within just a couple of days, I abandon my search for an apartment and decide to stay.

El Salam, the camp is called. Peace.

"Float with me," Katie calls from half a football field away.

We are snorkeling in the Red Sea. Well, Katie is, anyway. She dunks her head below the surface of the water. Her dreadlocks balance on the surface like tangled yellow yarn. Just when I think Katie has drowned, she pops back up again.

"Float with me!" she insists.

I cross my arms over my chest, hands holding on to my own sides, a rented snorkel mask hanging from my icy fingers. I am up to my knees in salty water.

"This water is freezing. The coral is cutting my feet. And god knows who used this snorkel before me," I say, gesturing with the chewed plastic mouthpiece.

Katie moves with the current, drifting forward and floating back again, a slender blonde scrap of seaweed on the tide. I understand why she has fish scales tattooed like a sleeve down her left arm.

"The water is clear and gorgeous. The coral is a marvel of nature. And someday you'll be far away from the Red Sea, and you'll regret not snorkeling with me," she laughs. "Come on. Last chance."

Before I can say anything, Katie submerges herself, legs kicking into the air. With toes pointed like a dancer, she snaps her ankles, and the rest of her body ripples like a cracked whip. She is gone.

I wait a few seconds before I call her name. I don't see any sign of her white snorkel tip or her ridiculously bright neon bathing suit.

I would head for the shore, but I don't want to be alone. I have no choice but to follow her.

I've always been terrible at judging distances, so I don't know how far I swim until I locate my friend again. Once reconnected, we swim a few dozen meters. Or maybe a few hundred. I don't know. The water is buoyant with salt, and even though I'm not a strong swimmer, I float easily.

We stop at a shallow reef, a popular dive site called Eel Garden. There the eels poke up through the sand, their curved shapes creating a field of underwater commas as they wait for the next meal to swim by.

"Let's give the eels a show," Katie says.

We giggle and take off our swimsuits, wrapping them around our wrists. Katie's bottoms float away and she kicks like mad to get to them before the waves abduct them forever. We imagine the bikini would wash up on the beach in Saudi Arabia, just across from us, where hardly anyone would know what it was. They might study it, build a glass case for it in a museum, make it the subject of a doctoral thesis.

"Swimming naked is the best," Katie says.

"It feels like I was just born," I say.

"Like nobody else exists," she says.

"Like nobody else *ever* existed," I add.

"Like the beginning of the world."

"Like the beginning of time."

We tread water for a few minutes then wade to the rocky beach, where I give Katie my towel to wrap around her waist. It is a clear evening. We see the lights turn on in Saudi Arabia.

Katie picks up stones and shows me how to grab brittle stars, long-limbed starfish about the size of our hands, from the shallow waters. Sometimes I scare them, and the legs fall off their starry button bodies.

My camera is in my bag, and I take photos of the sky emptying into the water, scoops of orange sherbet topped with petals of purple hyacinth. The colors unravel as we watch. This is the moment. The sunset is thick and ripe. A red streak slashes through the sky with a vivid gash. Salt water runs down my face.

I sit on the shore, knees curled to my chest, my shirt pulled over my legs. I cry, and Katie puts her head on my shoulder. Her hair tickles my sunburned neck.

"She's going right now," I whisper. "I just know it."

"You're probably right," Katie says. "And there's nothing you can do about it except wave goodbye."

She is correct. There is so much I want to do. There is nothing I can do.

I think about all those starfish I scared limbless. They're so vulnerable now. They don't even have the arms to flounder. It's enough to make me start crying again.

Katie grabs my hand and tugs me toward the boardwalk, which is lined with teahouses and Bedouin cafés. We can smell roasted chickens, sautéed garlic, boiled chickpeas laced with sumac. There are people everywhere. None of them are my mom.

Katie says she is so hungry she feels empty inside. I tell her to get used to it.

EGYPTIAN INTERNET SUCKS. I HAVE LITTLE ONLINE ACCESS at the yoga camp, and the Wi-Fi hotspots throughout Dahab are lukewarm at best.

I also don't have the cash to spend at a coffee shop if the free Wi-Fi isn't working. Instead I lean against a brick wall in an alley and piggyback on nearby unsecured networks with my iPhone. This has become my ritual, and I do it a few times a day.

Tonight I am more desperate than ever.

One connection lasts long enough to check my email, and I light a cigarette while I wait. Ever since my dad's message about my mom's declining health, I've been smoking, one of the dumbest things I can do with my asthma, but there's nobody to tell me to stop.

Connecting ... loading ...

I don't have any messages. I try to call, but nobody answers. My dad, my sister, my brother. All my calls head straight to voicemail. I don't want to leave a message.

That night I go to bed not knowing if my mom is alive or dead.

It is so cold; I pull my wool chullo hat from Peru over my ears. I stare at the white space of a yoga poster on the wall. I wait. The minutes are stretchy, hollow, and endless. The night is always longest for those who don't find sleep.

El Salam

—⸻—

IN THE MORNING, I FOREGO MY TYPICAL BACKPACKER breakfast of Nescafé, dry toast, and a plastic package of jam.

Today is special. Today I decide to eat at a real café, Bamboo House, a hangout for travelers thanks to the solid Wi-Fi connection. I walk past this place several times a day every day, often enough that the waiters greet me with local prices and a hearty *"Sabah el kheer!"*

The sweeping patio butts up against the craggy shoreline of the Red Sea, which this morning is placid and a cornflower blue. The café tables are inviting, and the smell of pastries is too good to ignore following such a long and lonely night.

I splurge on an Americano and lemon pancakes. The waiter, who also speaks English, is patient while I attempt to order in Arabic and fiercely butcher his language. As my order is prepared, I clear a space on the patio and plug in my netbook. The connection is quick and solid.

An email pops into my inbox swiftly. It's from my dad, and true to form, it's brief: "Margaret, I don't know if you know this, but mom passed away last night."

The pancakes are delivered. I burst into tears.

The waiter looks concerned. "Did you want honey pancakes? I thought you said lemon." I shake my head and wave him away.

It's all so stupid. The water is so blue. The sun is so bright. The lemon pancakes so sweet. Why hasn't the world stopped yet? Doesn't everybody know?

One thing that surprises me is how the news wounds me in an instant. After a decade of suffering alongside my mother, I assumed this end would come as a relief. It is supposed to be closure. That is the promise of an extended illness: it is a blessing when it ends.

Only now, here, in the eye of the moment, it is worse than I imagined. For all those years she was just out of reach, I carried a seed of hope. Now that hope will never grow into anything more.

I look around the Bamboo House patio, crowded with tourists from Europe and Russia. People with blond hair just like my mom. I know it's impossible that she would be here, but what if she came to me? What if she wanted to see me one last time? That sunset last night—was that it?

A weird cat with an astute gaze hops into my lap, and I ache for it to be some kind of sign, even though I'm sure it's not. My mom had two blue eyes, and this cat has one blue, one green.

I stroke the kitten, name him David Bowie, and feed him some of my pancakes. It's a win-win situation: I'm having trouble choking down food, and he is clearly hungry. His ribs heave as he chews.

"That cat's been hanging around forever," says one of the waiters. "His name is Ginger."

"But why? He's not ginger at all."

"It just is."

I want this to be meaningful, but I'm not sure how. I say this over and over again in my head: *It just is.*

I pay and leave. My instinct pushes me to wander, and I walk with no destination.

The man on the boardwalk who makes pictures of layered sand in bottles waves hello. I ignore him. I pass by Ghazala grocery store, a *koshary* stall,
incense shops, jewelry stores, a dozen *shisha* bars, and a souvenir hut called
Hump the Camel. There is a vendor who always points at my flip-flops and
says, "Nice socks!" I usually play along with him. Today I flip him off. What
a stupid fucking joke.

My mom is dead. My mom is dead. My mom is dead. I want to blast it
from the megaphones that broadcast prayers at the mosques. I want everybody to know.

I pass by a snorkeler waddling toward the water.

"My mom is dead!" I shout.

He nods his head in response.

I yell again, "I hope you drown!"

He smiles and waves.

It's difficult to go anywhere in Dahab without ending up back at the
Red Sea, so that's where I find myself again. I'm drawn to the edge, where
sea meets sand, and for a moment I think about walking straight in, letting
the water fill my pockets and tug me into the deep, testing how precarious life
can be. It is tempting in the way driving into oncoming traffic occasionally
seems tempting, not that I want to die, but I want to feel something different.

Eventually I turn away from the shore.

After some time my path leads me back to the yoga camp. The woman
who runs the place, an American named Dakini Runningbear, knows what
happened before I say anything. She's perceptive like that. Her arms open,
and I collapse into her brown hair, a tangle of sea salt and sand.

If you're going to have a mother who dies, El Salam is probably the best
place in the world to be when it happens. Word of my mother's death spreads
quickly through the dozen or so long-term residents, and they rush to take
on some of my pain.

Amy from England gets stoned and rubs my feet for an hour. Patrick
from Ireland gives me a package of black-market Valium. "You might need
this," he says, tucking the pills into my small backpack. Thomas from Den-
mark puts a sleepy kitten in my lap.

Dakini creates a makeshift latte by brewing espresso in a steel pot over a fire. She gingerly stirs the shot of caffeine into boiled camel milk and honey. It tastes fatty and salty sliding down my throat.

A German woman who calls herself The Gypsy Queen offers to do a tarot reading. We sit cross-legged on her bed, in a room that smells like smoke and cumin, sheer scarves hanging from the ceiling above. I don't remember most of what she says, but the reading lasts for what feels like hours.

Finally The Gypsy Queen instructs me to make a selection from a deck of "energy cards." I draw one that says "closure."

"Fuck you," I say to the card, and I leave her smelly room. The world has already given me closure, and it means my heart has been carved right out of my chest.

With nothing left to say, Katie and I set up a slackline between two palm trees. We take turns walking the tight rope and falling off, over and over again.

It was a cold day in Ohio. The schools were closed for snow. Swollen, pregnant clouds birthed gray into more gray. The wheat fields seemed flatter than usual. Ice hung from the skeletal trees.

A nurse called my dad at home and told him to come to the nursing home—it was the day. He and my sister each made the surreal drive down Interstate 675 toward a bland yellow room to watch a wife and mother die.

My mom's hair was long. Her cheeks were sunken. This woman who weighed 180 pounds in life didn't weigh more than 120 pounds at her death. She would have killed for that.

"She's going right now," the nurse told my dad.

My dad held my mother's hand. He looked to the floor and repeated, "Poor Heide. Poor, poor Heide." My sister stood behind the bed and stroked our mom's forehead, smoothing the hair from her face. A minister was a quiet shadow in the corner of the room.

Mom inhaled sharply for a few minutes, a hollow and raspy sound that shook the bones of everybody in the room.

"How long can we do this?" my sister asked.

Then mom quieted. Her body shuddered. She took a shallow breath and exhaled and then—

And then she was nothing anymore.

And then I no longer had a mom.

"That's it?" my dad said.

My dad and my sister thanked the minister. They packed up my mom's things, erasing every sign of her from the nursing home room. They drove home the same way they arrived. Separately.

THE KING CHICKEN DELIVERY BOY ARRIVES AT THE YOGA camp at night carrying two bags of dog food. The sacks weigh about ten kilos each and contain the restaurant's dinner scraps—chicken bones and skin, fat and cartilage, potato peels and greasy napkins, even the occasional plastic fork.

The delivery boy is a baby-faced teen named Ali. Sometimes he brings lunch, sometimes he brings dog food, and the bags look identical. I've been a resident at the yoga camp long enough that he and I are familiar.

Tonight Ali slings the bags over the camp's fence, then empties them into heaps on the floor near the kitchen. While a dozen dogs fight over chicken bones, Ali sinks into one of the outdoor couches where my makeshift yoga family drinks watery Egyptian beer and lights a hookah filled with apple-flavored tobacco.

I don't return Ali's smile. He asks why. I tell him my mom died, and I explain she suffered from a terrible disease for many years.

"She was very old?" he says.

"Seventy."

"Ah, long life," Ali nods.

"Not long enough."

Ali says in Egypt, people are lucky to reach such an admirable old age. That might be true. But when Ali says she went to a better place, I disagree. I don't know if I believe there is a better place.

"It doesn't matter what you believe," he says. "*Inna lillah hi wa inna ilaihi rajioon.* To him we belong and to him we shall return."

"But I don't want her to return," I say. I slide my blue plastic flip-flop off my foot and draw lines in the dirt with my toes. "I'm selfish."

I suppose I imagined my mom would disappear from my life with swiftness. A car accident. A heart attack. Something understandable, something I could wrap my head around. But having her taken this way, in a prolonged state of grief, has been overwhelming. She was an elegant woman claimed by something completely undignified. There is no reason for it. Certainly no god would do this.

Ali gives me a hug. "Old people have to die to make room for the young people to get old. It's better this way."

We sit this way for a long time: Me, body crumpled, eyes closed. Him, a thirteen-year-old kid draped around my shoulders. The night is quiet except for waves slapping against the coast. The sky is crammed with stars and billows of smoke.

My head is heavy with thought and soggy with uncried tears. I can't even articulate if I am sad or angry or confused or fatigued. I am a mix of things. I am furiously sad. I am angrily exhausted.

As a newspaper reporter, I was acquainted with destruction. I've seen bodies twisted in metal and shards of wreckage. I've watched the arduous process of pulling a decomposing body from the Ohio River. I've witnessed morticians draining fluids, sewing mouths closed, and pasting rough contact lenses over lifeless eyeballs to snag the eyelids and keep them shut. I've seen enough death to know that a body is not a person. It is a life edited down to a pocketful of words: Heide-Marie Downs, born August 30, 1940, died January 12, 2011.

I know what is happening to my mom's body now. I know that what I loved was long gone. I know she descended into dementia while I was still an awful person doing regrettable things, and she will never enjoy the person I've become, because death is so frustrating and final. I know I feel something for the first time in years, and I am desperate to stop this ferocious emptiness.

Ali breaks the silence.

"Hey, you got any weed?" he says.

That's when I begin to cry, abruptly injected into my own story again: Rocked by the skinny but heavy arms of a boy. The sound of wild dogs crushing chicken bones. A night sky so close it suffocates me.

THE DRIVER PICKS ME UP AROUND 3 A.M.

Abdullah is confident and lifts my duffel bag without asking if I want him to carry it. He walks purposefully, a quick apparition through the cobblestone streets, forcing me to move faster to keep pace. The grubby drunks wilting against stairwells and low-slung doorways wave hello, and Abdullah responds with an economical nod of the head.

The lanky Bedouin wears a long galabeya robe topped by a leather bomber jacket to ward off the slithery Red Sea wind. A gold-and-ivory *shemagh* wraps his head like a coiled snake.

There is no apprehension in my step as I follow him into the dark alleys. He is a friend of Dakini Runningbear's Bedouin boyfriend, and I know he will take care of me. They say Bedouins are loyal, and I've seen nothing to disprove that. I also know that Abdullah is charming—Dakini once said he could steal the mascara off a woman's eyes—but I don't wear mascara, so there is nothing to steal.

Inside the car, Abdullah blasts the heat, then fiddles with a cheap knock-off MP3 player called a yPod. He switches between Akon and the Eagles.

"Which you need?" he says gently.

I shake my head. I don't want either. He settles on the Eagles, the song where you can check out anytime you like but you can never leave.

"Drink?" he says, handing me a sweating box of guava juice. I take it from him, grateful. I am drained and thirsty.

I had wrestled with the idea of flying home for the funeral, and I came up with a hundred reasons why I shouldn't. My mom was in Ohio. I was on the other side of the world. My family said I shouldn't come. It was expensive. It wasn't practical. I lost her many years ago. Funerals aren't important.

There was no point. She is dead. She is dead. She is dead. I made peace with my decision to stay in Egypt.

But I couldn't shake the tug to go. My mom would never know I was there, but I would. After a couple of clicks at the internet café and one call to my travel insurance, I had a hastily packed duffel bag and a plane ticket to Columbus, Ohio.

I purposely kept my big blue backpack at the yoga camp to give myself a reason to return eventually. I know myself well, and I know how easy it would be to fold under my grief, become complacent, stay home. I need to keep going with whatever this trip is—I think that's what my mom would have wanted. The only possible way to move on is to keep moving.

Just a handful of hours later, I am in Abdullah's car, barreling through an inky desert to the airport in Sharm el-Sheikh.

We arrive far too early. It is near four in the morning, and my flight doesn't leave until seven. I can't even check in for two more hours. I imagine my short-term future will involve bumming cigarettes off strangers and shivering in front of the terminal.

Abdullah pulls his car off the road, within sight of the airport but too far to walk, and puts the vehicle into park. Terror jolts through me. An instinct. My muscles tense to a point of trembling.

"Stay," Abdullah says, a voice as rough as shrapnel.

He yanks the handle on the side of my seat, causing it to snap backward. Abdullah leans close, and I am intimate with his fleshy, musky cologne. The car feels small. He is practically crouched on top of me as he works to slip the bomber jacket off his shoulders. I am too frightened to move. We are alone. Screaming would be pointless. I have let my guard down, and I have no idea what the consequences will be.

Abdullah wads his jacket into a ball, then gingerly slips his hand behind my head to lift it and places the jacket softly like a pillow.

"It's not time yet," he whispers, returning to his seat on the driver's side. "First you must sleep."

My muscles soften and ooze back into place. I realize he already knows why I am in his car and why I'm headed to the airport. Abdullah twists all the air vents toward me for optimum heat, then turns down the yPod and selects a slow song. When it begins to play, he clears his throat and warbles along.

This Bedouin is a Celine Dion fan. This fact is made clear over the next two hours as I drift in and out of sleep to a soundtrack of her biggest hits, accompanied by Abdullah's smoky accent. It envelops me, surprisingly soothing and comforting, even though I am no fan.

When it is time, Abdullah nudges me awake. "Miss Maggie, you must go home," he says.

It doesn't take long to trudge through security lines and board my flight. The plane lifts into the air, the aircraft squeezing out from under the blanched, overcast sky into the space where morning is born again. Out the window I watch as the sun splits open, a runny egg spilling over the clouds, the wing, my face.

LIFE

God it's great to be alive
Takes the skin right off my hide
To think I'll have to give it all up someday.

—DANIEL JOHNSTON

A Revolution Begins

"Just a quick phone call," my dad said, and he handed me a folded twenty-dollar bill to purchase an international calling card. His forehead was furrowed with worry, his wispy hair more gray than it had ever been before. "Just to let me know you're safe."

Those were his parting words to me when I left Ohio, one week after my mom's funeral. Now I've landed in Cairo, and my only mission is to call home.

In the airline terminal, I walk past a bank of pay phones, all of them unused. I stuff my hand in my pocket and feel for the plastic calling card I bought at JFK during my layover. With it in hand, I stop at one of the phones. When I pick it up, the line is dead. I shift to the next phone and pick up the receiver. That one is dead too. Same with the next. And the one after that. All the phones, dead.

I know there's an internet café in the airport, so I head that direction. If I can't call, at least I can Skype or send my family an email. My dad is at home alone with a weak and sad heart, still unmoored and mourning, and I know he's waiting to hear that I've arrived here safely. I want to ease his worry as much as I can. Without my mom at the nursing home, I am his focus now.

Clusters of people push past, a collection of black and gray hijabs, swishy caftans, sandals that whisper "ship-ship-ship" with each step. Nobody seems to understand the gravity of my situation; everybody looks to the space beyond me.

The internet café is closed, a handwritten Arabic note on the locked door. I can't read it, but I assume it's a routine down-for-maintenance kind of message. This country has the worst internet.

At the information desk in the airport's main lobby, I ask if there's another place to hop online. The woman working at the desk sets her mouth in a line.

"No," she says. "Bad day for internet."

"So all the internet is down?"

"Yes," she says. "Bad day."

When I turn away from the desk, it's the first time I notice the men stationed in the windows. The entrance of the Cairo airport is all light and glass, like facets of a gemstone, with windows that begin halfway up the wall and soar to the ceiling. The men are in uniform, long-sleeve black shirts and pants, perched on the windowsills, holding automatic weapons. The way they are positioned—arms locked, legs wide, weapons at the ready—they look like toys, like plastic army men arranged in a row.

There are more uniformed men on the ground. They wear crisp white outfits, like sea captains.

I pivot toward the information desk and ask the woman, "What's happening?" She shrugs.

My eye catches a TV playing BBC News. The headline flashes bold red letters on the screen: "EGYPT IN CRISIS!"

I gasp when I see the chyron, and I half expect someone to pop out on the screen and say it's all a joke. How can Egypt be in crisis? I've only been gone less than two weeks.

All I want is to return to the same Egypt that supported me when I suffered, the same Egypt where I discovered arms to hold me at a yoga camp, the Egypt of ancient ruins and fresh kindness.

Except it isn't the same place.

My intention was to stay in Cairo for a few days and grieve here. I had hoped to return to the tombs in Giza, where I could mourn my mom among the long dead, the people who believed death was only a temporary interruption to life. Instead I find turmoil greater than what I am feeling internally, and I don't know what to do. I don't know what's happening, and I don't feel equipped to make any decisions.

I should go directly to my hostel in Tahrir Square, I think. But on my way out the door of the airport, a guard yanks me by the shoulder and stops me.

"Don't stay in Cairo," he says. "It's better to go."

There's a grave quality to his voice, and it's enough to turn me around. I need a safe and orderly place—I thought that's what I was doing by returning to Cairo—but if the universe has proven anything over the past month, it has disabused me of the illusion of control.

I buy a ticket to Sharm el-Sheikh to make my way back to Dahab, back to my friends at the yoga camp, and back to the place where I stashed my backpack. Within a couple of hours, I'm on board another plane. I don't know what waits for me in Dahab or how dangerous the situation might become. I have no choice but to find out.

Take the Hash

THE ARAB SPRING IGNITES QUICKLY AND FIERCELY. PRO-
testors throughout the country demand the resignation of President Hosni
Mubarak, and the air is restless. I am restless.

The government has shut off the internet, and phone access is limited.
The lack of information unravels me. I know my family must be frantic. I still
haven't been able to contact them. I pace the streets of Dahab, a zoo animal
caged in the wrong habitat. I start running again, just to burn off my stress.

Within just a couple of days, all the ATMs in town run dry. I try to use
them anyway. Jason has access to all of my bank information, and I hope my
account will show every attempt to use a bank machine. An attempt means
I am alive.

A week later Dahab is feeling the effects from shortages of food, drinking water, and fuel, and I am skeptical about my chances of getting out of
the country if the situation escalates. Will the situation escalate? Without
news or internet, it's hard to gauge. I focus on my stockpile of granola bars

and instant-oatmeal packets, too anxious about my own life to grieve my mother's death.

Dakini Runningbear believes there is only one way to steady our trembling spirits—more yoga, more stretches, more deep breaths into the places that hurt.

She asks us to set an intention for nurturing and growth, for peace to blossom in between the cracks of the cement in Cairo. We practice yoga outside in the sun for hours upon hours, executing our postures to a soundtrack of "Rock the Casbah" and the Beatles' "Revolution." There's an Egyptian heavy metal band staying at the camp now too, unable to return to Cairo during the chaos, and they join us in the yoga classes.

"Let your muscles release healing energy into the world," Dakini says brightly, and that is what I try to do.

For the first time since I started doing yoga, my tree pose falters. My leg is wobbly, my body unsteady, and I tip over, bruising my hand when I try to catch myself. I'm neither strong nor stable. There's no way I can withstand a revolution; I can't even stand.

When I try to buy a bus ticket out of town, I'm told there are no buses running. Try again in a week. My friends at the yoga camp tell me to relax, and I find that impossible. It might be different if I could contact my family, but the lack of communication makes me frantic. My anxiety is at an all-time high. Who knows how long the revolution will last?

I count my dwindling stash of granola bars and instant-oatmeal packets. I don't have much food left. A week's worth, maybe. With the lack of grocery deliveries to the Sinai Peninsula, the situation feels like it could turn bad fast. My friends have stockpiled some food as well, mostly sacks of flatbread and canned beans, but they are confident the situation will resolve soon, and they are not worried. They encourage me to stay. They say we are safer together. My friends are prepared to weather this storm, to stay and fight. I have no fight left to give.

Abdullah, my Celine Dion–loving driver, offers to bring me to the port town of Nuweiba, where I can safely flee Egypt. I say yes. His Bedouin status means we can leave after dark, long past the government-imposed evening curfew, and we leave that night.

We travel in a white Jeep, the only speck of lightness on a black desert road. Whenever we encounter police checkpoints, Abdullah hands them juice boxes and cigarettes. They smile and wave us on.

We stop at a Bedouin camp on the seashore just outside of Nuweiba. It is late, and I am disoriented. The air is briny, the night wind howling. This is where Abdullah will leave me with Hakeem, his friend who owns the camp, a chain-smoking man with the face of a prune.

We sit cross-legged around a bonfire near the sea, propped up on soggy pillows. Abdullah spreads out dinner—bread shaped like hot dog buns, processed cheese cubes in foil, a snack-sized bag of potato chips, and canned fruit cocktail. Before we eat, Abdullah smiles and says, "*Baynana aish wamilah.*" Between us, bread and salt.

He says this is a popular proverb in Egypt, and it means that if I have broken bread with you, I trust you. We have nourished ourselves at the same table. Therefore, there can be no fighting, no animosity between us. There will only be goodness.

When we are done eating, we watch the moon, ripe and tangerine, paint silky ripples of water. The wind has calmed, and the night is clear. On the other side of the sea is a city where I will hopefully be tomorrow, and the lights glitter like jewels on a chain. Somewhere there I'll buy a cell phone and stack it full of minutes and hear the relief in my dad's voice. I'll call my husband and tell him I love him. Such a simple dream, but it feels like a distant one.

Abdullah leaves to boil water for drinking. Hakeem speaks to me for the first time all night.

"May I ask you a question?" he says.

"Of course."

"What is a period?"

"It is a dot at the end of a sentence," I say. "It means that something has come to an end."

"No, no," he corrects me. "*Woman* period. What is woman period?"

How do you describe your body to a stranger?

I got my period for the first time when I was thirteen, visiting my sister who at the time lived in Minot, North Dakota. We were supposed to visit the missile fields to tour a nuclear silo, crammed with warheads. Instead I went to the restroom that morning and found blood on my underwear.

My family thought it would be best for me to stay behind, so my mom, my dad, my sister, and her husband left without me. I stayed on the couch, alternating between swells of pride and terror at what my body could do, the things my body could contain—something as miraculous as it was devastating. It was life made very real.

"Some people call it 'moon time,'" I say. "They say this is a sacred time for women, when we release our old energy and prepare to reconnect with our fertile power."

Hakeem contemplates this for a moment and then says he doesn't understand, which of course he doesn't. I was saying words but not explaining anything at all. I look to the Red Sea and stifle a laugh. This sounds like the setup for a terrible joke.

"Sometimes, um . . . women . . . bleed. Here," I wave my hand in a circle above my abdomen.

"Ah, yes," Hakeem nods. "This is why women are eaten by sharks."

I grab a cigarette from Hakeem's pack and disguise the awkward silence with quick puffs of smoke.

Hakeem, however, won't let the conversation rest. He makes ugly declarations about women. "Men don't bleed unless they are injured," he says. "This period is proof God hates women. He makes women weak and pitiful. Women get what they deserve. You are just blood."

His face is distorted by the bonfire flames. In the flickering shadows, his hairy, wrinkly face looks half-man, half-testicle. I toss the rest of my cigarette into the fire and watch it burn.

I think about how I rearranged the parts of my life for this moment. How I quit my job to venture around the world. How I flew 8,000 miles to be with my broken family. How I left my mom in the hard, January earth and continued wandering the world, in search of something I can't yet articulate.

I thought I had a clear reason for making this journey, but now that my mom is gone, I'm not sure anymore.

Those words echo: *You are just blood.* I believe I am far more than my blood—although isn't that the reason I am traveling? If I don't have this blood connecting me to my ancestors, what else do I have? It is this blood ripping through my veins right now that keeps me alive and vibrant and seeking. It is also this blood that might become my undoing, the genetic curse that might one day steal my memory. This blood is my inheritance.

I say none of these things to Hakeem. I just hate him.

When Abdullah returns, he walks me to a cluster of low huts. I hear lapping water nearby and faraway gunshots.

"Abdullah, I'm scared."

"You will be safe," he says. He props my backpack against one hut and unrolls several rugs on the sand, making a bed for me to sleep.

"Abdullah, I hear gunshots."

"Oh, not gunshots. This is Bedouins playing and dancing." He stretches his index fingers out like pistols and fires them into the air. "Ha ha ha! Bang bang bang. Is just for fun."

I appreciate that he cares enough to lie. It's something my mom would have done.

Abdullah leaves me with presents: Three packages of Nescafé instant cappuccino. One package of chocolate cookies. The shemagh scarf that was wrapped around his head. When I bring it to my nose, it smells of sandalwood mixed with something slightly Camaro-y, like the Egyptian version of Drakkar Noir.

He also hands me a fat bag of hash.

"I don't want to cross any borders with this," I say.

"Trust me," he says.

There is only the slightest door on my hut, a thin sheet of plywood that doesn't fully close. I point to it, and Abdullah takes my hand in his. "Trust me," he says again before he leaves for good.

And I do. Between us, bread and salt. Abdullah is my bread, warm and comforting. Hakeem is salt, unpalatable in large doses. Both necessary.

I wake up just a few feet from this biblical sea, where Moses helped the slaves escape from Egypt, where I was told God hates women. I walk to the edge of the seashore and scrub my face with briny water. From here I can see the rusty mountains of Saudi Arabia, the faraway coast of Jordan, the smallest sliver of Israel. I wade in knee-deep, half hoping the water will part for me.

As the sea laps around my legs, I think about how I interpreted my wobbly tree pose all wrong. It's not that I am too weak to remain; it's that I am flexible enough to kiss the ground and stand again. I bend without breaking.

Hakeem drives me to the port two hours before the ferry is scheduled to leave. He offers to carry my backpack during the short walk to a roadside café, where he sits me down at a plastic table. He hugs my backpack and says he will hold it for ransom until I give him 1,000 American dollars.

It's a preposterous request, and I'm not frightened by it. As a journalist, I have endured anthrax scares, death threats, and stalkers. When I wrote an article about a high school football coach who gave teenage girls gifts of lingerie, I arrived home to find one of the coach's supporters waiting on my porch with a shotgun. A Mother's Day column prompted a reader to fill my voicemail with a rant about how she wanted me to die of Alzheimer's. Every week for one year, I received unsigned postcards that contained a single word: "cunt." I am an inadvertent expert in determining which threats are real and which ones are noise. I know how to diffuse anger, to be accommodating, to bite my tongue.

I don't have the money Hakeem wants. Because the ATMs are empty, I have only enough for the ferry ride, maybe a couple of Egyptian pounds more. I wouldn't give him $1,000 anyway. I'd rather walk away from my things and leave Hakeem holding the remnants of a woman who was too strong to stay.

Instead I give him the bag of hash. This makes him happy, and he shouts out orders for food.

We are served French fries, falafel, and *fuul*, a dish of slow-cooked fava beans with tomatoes, onions, and swirls of tahini. Hakeem tears a piece of pita in two and hands me half, and I use it to mop up the fuul. It is delicious and salty, only slightly bitter. When it comes time to leave for Jordan, I don't even wave goodbye.

Room for More

⸻⸺⸻

My introduction to Petra is by night.

The narrow gorge that leads to the ancient city's ruins runs nearly a mile, like an artery that pumps people toward the heart of the place. It is called the *siq*, and it's a fault in the earth, ripped apart by tectonic forces. When the Nabatean capital city of Petra was established around 312 BC, this was the grand caravan entrance, traveled by merchants, traders, and Roman soldiers. Archeological evidence suggests this was also a sacred space.

Tonight the siq is lit by tea lights that illuminate the canyon walls with an ethereal glow. Overhead I see a smattering of stars.

These looming walls should be enough to terrify me. They are tall—up to 600 feet high in some places—and it is dark. A Bedouin guide has asked everyone making this journey to go in silence, so the only sound comes from echoing footsteps and the occasional braying donkey and mewling cat. But the siq comforts me in the idea that something that has been ruthlessly split apart could continue to pulse with life.

I wonder how many mothers have passed through these stones over the

years, how many families traveled here for food or water or spiritual sustenance. Hundreds of thousands, maybe even millions of people whom I will
never know, their names lost to the past. All roads lead to this place—where
voices, names, and blood disappear into the earth—and still the world stands,
holding fast to these secrets.

The passage opens up at Al Khazneh, the Treasury, Petra's most recog-
nizable building. It's an elaborate structure carved out of the rosy sandstone
rock, built sometime in the first century. It is also one of the final things on
my mom's list.

Tonight the Treasury glows red with candles. Rugs are arranged on the
desert floor, and people from all over the world squat or sit cross-legged. Bedouin musicians play songs and sing in lilting Arabic. I can't understand a
single word, but every one of them seems to slice right through to my heart.
I close my eyes and sway. Each time I inhale, the sharp desert smell reminds
me of my California home—the green scent of herbal plants, the subtle but
solid aroma of arid earth.

Though the Arab Spring continues to swirl around the Middle East, I
have safely evacuated Egypt, and I am in a stable place. I'm also with people I know. On the ferry from Egypt to Jordan, I ran into Rose and Hew,
friends from Dahab, and we are traveling together for a bit.

As soon as the ferry made it to Aqaba, we found a hostel with Wi-Fi, and
I contacted my family for the first time in almost two weeks. I didn't even
know what time it was in Ohio; I only knew the call would be answered.

"Dad?"

"Oh, Margaret, Margaret, Margaret," he said. His voice broke at the
sound of mine, until it splintered into a wail. "Come home. Why won't you
come home?"

My dad was never one to express his feelings, but that night, before we
hung up the phone, he said he loved me.

Next I called Jason, who knew I was alive—he had been following the
electronic trail of ATM withdrawals—and I reassured him that I would
carefully follow the news and stay safe.

Nobody wants me to stay in Jordan. My family believes an uprising in

one Middle Eastern country will become an uprising in every country, but I
don't want to leave. Not yet. I feel the presence of my mom here in the sweep
of desert, the shifting sands, the streaky rock formations.

I remember a road trip we took out West when I was about twelve or
thirteen years told. My sister and brother were already adults and had moved
away from home, so it was just my dad, my mom, and me, together for a couple of weeks in a maroon Buick. We departed Ohio and followed part of the
Oregon Trail, stopping in dusty, sweltering towns along the way, then looped
around to South Dakota, through Badlands National Park. Our goal was to
reach Mount Rushmore, but I discovered the Badlands were the true marvel.

It spoke to me in a way that no landscape ever had before. I took dozens
of photos—and this was before we had a digital camera—so I clicked and
filled frame after frame of bizarre outcroppings, sharp spires, and layers of
eroded strata. I was enchanted by all of it. The ombré of color. The desolation and melancholy. It's a place where you can't tell the difference between
what's breaking down and what's rising up, but either one creates a sense of
possibility.

"Isn't it amazing?" I gasped. My mom agreed and laced her fingers
through mine. I thought I was too old for holding my mother's hand, but I
let it go this one time, since nobody was around to see us. We were quiet for a
moment as we gazed across the expanse. Then I broke the silence.

"Why do you think they called this the Badlands?"

"Because the Goodlands would sound silly," she said.

It was a joke (the Lakota tribe gave the land its name, "Mako Sica," which
means "land bad"), but I can't help thinking of it now, surrounded by another rugged and breathtaking landscape. I am far from the "goodlands" of
my childhood, separated by distance and time from the place where I stood
in awe and held my mother's hand.

What I wouldn't give to hold her hand again. What I wouldn't give to
make space for her on this rug, to sit by the dancing candlelight in this monument of carved rock and empty tombs, to let the low and primal hum of the
music move through us.

My eyes are wet as I look around this magical spot. The canyons and rocks here are a consolation, an assurance that it's possible to weather time and tragedy and still be a thing of formidable beauty.

Finally, I mourn. This ancient place holds my sadness too.

I SPEND THE NEXT DAY AT PETRA, CLAMBERING OVER THE canyons, hiking through the ruins, experiencing the city from every possible vantage point. Petra Archeological Park was declared a UNESCO World Heritage Site in 1985. Archaeologists speculate that only a small portion of the city has been uncovered, but what's there is spectacular.

After a full day of sightseeing, I return to the town of Wadi Musa, where I'm staying in a hostel for the night. Abraham, one of the owners, invites me to join him and his friends for an authentic Jordanian dinner.

Abraham negotiates his Land Cruiser through narrow side streets of the congested city, barely missing a pack of small children and grazing donkeys. We speed past handwritten Arabic signs, crumbling homes, and shops made of sagging wood. Soon we are past the limits of town and out in the mountainous desert. I'm in the backseat with a man on either side, their faces ruddy and chapped by wind.

"So where are we going?" I ask.

"You'll see," Abraham says. He flicks his lighter, singes the end of his Dunhill cigarette, and puffs at it. His friends joke in Arabic. I can pluck out a word or two, but most of the conversation floats past me.

There are no more roads, at least none that I can discern. Dusk buckles under the darkness, and soon we're traveling through a canvas of ebony sky. A half hour later, the vehicle groans to a stop on a blank swath of desert, populated only by a few scrubby bushes and jagged rock formations. Shortly after we arrive, another vehicle pulls up and parks near us.

"When you said we were going out to eat, I thought you meant a restaurant down the street," I say. "I didn't know you meant *outside*."

He laughs. "It's cool," he says. "This is Jordan barbecue."

I don't even know how that's possible here. There is nothing to barbecue on—no kitchen, no grill, not even a source of heat.

"*Yalla*," Abraham says, and his friends scatter. They return within moments with branches, handfuls of twigs, and one dry, dead tree. A few of the guys construct a fire pit—a hole in the ground into which they place a metal rack—while another pulls supplies from the trunk. Abraham readies the food. My offers to help are brushed aside.

When the fire has mostly settled into hot coals, Abraham buries the food inside. Eggplants and a head of garlic are positioned under the embers. Chicken and roughly sliced onions go on the rack.

Ahab, a lanky guy in his early twenties, spears dozens of raw chicken legs on a metal rack and hoists the meat into the air triumphantly.

"Look at me! I am hunter!" and his friends cheer.

The chicken is rubbed with fresh greens and a fragrant spice mix, then balanced over the fire. A layer of potatoes, wrapped in wet cloth, is placed on the top shelf of the rack. Ahab spreads two blankets over the opening of the pit; then another friend shovels sand over the blankets. This will take hours to cook, and my stomach is already grumbling.

As we wait, Abraham puts the key in the ignition to start the car radio. I expect something traditionally Jordanian. What I get is Jack Johnson.

"Is this like being in California?" Abraham smiles as the song "Bubble-toes" plays. His hair is long and unruly, flopping over his eyes as he talks. He dances a little bit to the song and sings along.

"Kind of," I laugh. "Okay, not really. I've never cooked my food outside in the desert like this."

The truth is, this could be California—or any number of places I've found around the world. These are the essential ingredients for every gathering in every culture, everywhere. Friends, food, music. They are the building blocks of almost every memory I have too.

When I think about my mom, she's often in the kitchen making supper, bent over the sink or a cutting board when a song she likes comes on the radio. She wipes a hand on a dish towel, turns up the volume, and shakes her hips to the beat. Then she gestures to me to join in. That's how I remember it, anyway: laughter and singing, unraveling the day with joyful, uninhibited dancing. Perhaps that's not the truth of it—maybe not every evening of my childhood was a spontaneous dance party—but that's how it lives in my head.

"Take a plate," Abraham says.

He digs the eggplant from the ashes and plops the vegetable on a plate. The charred skin peels off in one satisfying layer. The garlic cloves are now roasted and squishy, and Abraham squashes a few of them onto the eggplant. He adds a dollop of yogurt and a pinch of salt, slices a lemon in half and squeezes the juice over the entire plate. Then he mashes everything together with a fork before adding a generous drizzle of olive oil. He tears a piece of bread and dredges it through the mixture, then offers it to me.

I've eaten eggplant but never like this. It is smoky and creamy, with a depth of flavor I've never tasted before. He gives me another piece of bread, and I scoop the mixture greedily. After nearly two weeks of stale granola bars and instant oatmeal, the taste of a homemade meal is something akin to love.

It fills my stomach quickly, but Abraham laughs and says I can surely eat forty more bites.

The metal rack is retrieved from the fire pit. Potatoes are split open and sprinkled with salt. There's a platter of blackened chicken and heaps of salad. We eat lentils and rice, tomatoes and cucumbers, bread smeared with garlic and oil.

I lose track of how many hours we spend warming our hands over a fire, coaxing down warm beers, singing and passing plates around. Every time I think I'm full, somehow there's room for more.

The Only Way Out Is Through

IT'S MID-FEBRUARY 2011, WELL INTO MY SEVENTH MONTH of travel, and I'm in Addis Ababa, wandering the halls of the National Museum of Ethiopia. The basement here is home to the partial skeleton of Lucy, a 3.2-million-year-old ancestor to humans found in the northwestern Afar region of Ethiopia. She was named Lucy because "Lucy in the Sky with Diamonds" played on a cassette tape while paleontologists excavated her bones from the dirt, which feels whimsical considering she's also known as the grandmother of humanity.

It has been nearly one month since my mom died, and though I have felt the bracing immediacy of that loss every day, I am finally becoming acquainted with the depths of my sorrow.

The Arab Spring distracted me in Egypt with fear, stress, and anxiety. Alternatively, Jordan was a distracting relief, where I could while away my time with sightseeing and keep myself occupied with new friends.

What I discover in Ethiopia is that distracting myself from pain doesn't mean dissolving the pain. I've been walking the streets, hoping the movement would somehow pull me away from myself, but it's as futile as outrunning a shadow. Everywhere I go, there I am. And what I am is furiously sad.

Barbara is supposed to meet me here later in the month, and we will travel to the southern countryside together; until she arrives, I am alone with my pain.

I thought this museum would at least give me something pretty to look at, but all it's done is make me think about family, ancestry, and the bones we leave behind. It's not lost on me that Ethiopia marks time by a Julian calendar, made up of twelve months of thirty days, plus another month of just five days. That means the years here don't pass at the same rate as they do with a Western calendar. So it's 2011 for most of the world, but I walk through Addis Ababa in 2003. Present me is here, but I am stuck in the past.

There is a ritual aspect to death, and that part is comforting. Everyone since Lucy has participated in this. It is something my great-grandparents did, then my grandparents. My mom simply followed suit. Someday I will do it too.

Why then do endings feel so gutting?

In this moment, I think it's because I am alone, and I am steeped in it. Distracting myself from grief didn't work, and distance hasn't helped either. My only choice now is to go through it, which is where I am now, and nobody else can join me in this place.

A security guard stops me as I make my way out of the Lucy room.

"Are you alone?" he says.

All I can do is nod.

Traveling Ethiopia is hard. The first time I try to retrieve money from an ATM, my bank cancels my Visa. My backup is a MasterCard, which is not accepted in this country.

It's a long, convoluted process for my husband to wire cash, which he does, but the fees are steep, and my hostel charges interest on every night's stay and every meal that I can't immediately pay. When my hostel runs out of water, I don't have the ability to go anywhere else until I obtain more money.

Then one last devastation: a new editor at the newspaper in Palm Springs, which has been running my travel articles on a freelance basis, says he no longer needs my work.

Some of the street beggars have been aggressive, and twice I am pinned against a building by men demanding money. I have nothing to give.

The unfortunate thing is that Ethiopia is one of the places I was looking forward to the most. It is a place of stunning natural beauty, from the lakes and lush grasses of the Rift Valley to the rugged Semien Mountains. The carved churches of Lalibela, the crater lakes and sulfur springs of the Danakil Depression, and the palaces of Gondar are like nothing else on this planet. Also the food is extraordinary. Most meals revolve around stews served on injera, which looks like a limp pancake made out of fermented teff flour and tastes like spongy sourdough. The food is eaten with your hands, tearing pieces of injera to sop up the sloppy beans and curries, so it engages every sense, right down to the steamy sauna of sauce sliding down your fingertips.

There are beautiful things to be found here, I know this to be true. But I am still far gone in a pit of desolation, and every difficulty I encounter in the capital city sends me spiraling farther down.

After about a week, I get to a point that everyday horrors barely register. I feel mechanical. Case in point: I don't even notice the dying donkey on the sidewalk until after I step over him. Only afterward do I turn around and offer a second glance.

I'm with Tanya, a friend I met in Rwanda, whom I had the good fortune of running into again in Ethiopia. She's an Australian social worker, traveling the continent of Africa with her husband, Paul, in a Land Cruiser with a pop-up tent.

Tanya stops, presses her hands against her heart, and makes sympathetic noises. This is one of the things that drew me to her from the start—her heart is almost too big for her body. She can't tear her eyes away from the suffering animal.

The donkey's gray fur is matted with sweat, urine, and dirt. Chunks of skin have been torn from the length of his legs, leaving behind a red rawness, something more akin to animal flesh in the butcher shop. Pink lesions dot his trembling mouth, and his eyes weep pus and tears. He pants. His ear flicks. He appears to be about one inhale away from never breathing again.

We walk on. There is nothing we can do.

A few minutes later, Tanya turns around and tugs me back toward the donkey. His form is completely motionless. I shake my head and turn away. We are too late, and I don't have the emotional capacity for more death.

Tanya pulls a plastic grocery bag and a bottle of water from her backpack. She situates the bag underneath the donkey's snout, careful to avoid covering his nostrils, and pours a small bit of water inside the bag. The donkey's eyelids flutter.

While the donkey no longer has the energy to move his head, the side of his mouth tries to slurp the water. Slowly, slowly, he licks the puddle of water dry. Again, Tanya fills the plastic bag with water and tips it enough to drain into the donkey's mouth.

By now a small crowd has formed around us. People who had been hurrying to catch the bus, vendors from local stalls, women with babies in their arms, taxi drivers, businessmen—they all stop. One man says the donkey has been there for three days, but this is the first time anyone has stopped and offered help.

Tanya and I carefully hoist the donkey's head and neck up a few inches to give him a better angle for drinking. One leg kicks. Then another.

"Water makes donkey strong!" says a man on the street, who had paused to watch the commotion.

Another man walks along the sidewalk and picks handfuls of grass and weeds. He brings these greens to the donkey and lays them beside the animal's head. Two more men lift the donkey a few inches off the ground, then position him a few feet away on flatter, less rocky ground.

"It's better," one man says, nodding his head to the donkey. "More comfort."

By this time, the donkey has guzzled nearly four liters of water and looks remarkably better. He doesn't have the ability to stand on his own, but he no longer looks pained either. While I pet the donkey, Tanya looks up the number for a donkey-rescue organization—because those exist in Ethiopia—then calls and instructs them on how to find the animal.

I don't know how long the donkey will live. But Tanya's compassion shows me how action snowballs into inspiration, which in turn becomes a call to action for others. Where people were moving about on the street in their daily lives, suddenly they were willing to help another creature. Where I thought there was nothing I could do for another living being, there was.

What horrifies me most about the incident isn't the dying donkey but my initial indifference. Who am I in this world if I can't stoop to give water to a suffering creature? What else do we have if not each other?

It makes me wonder what else I could have given to my mother in the years she spent dying. I remember visiting the nursing home after she had been living there for a year. She was hunched over in a wheelchair, curled forward, her head drooped against her chest. I stroked her fine gray hair back and called, "Mom?" She never looked up at me. She never met my gaze. And it didn't make any sense, why she was still there. Why she mattered to the world.

Tanya and I continue down the street wordlessly. She's lost in her own thoughts. Meanwhile I struggle to figure out why my mom's spirit stubbornly remained for so long and what purpose that served. Why the donkey was still kicking when it had every right to give up.

Deep in the Omo Valley, inside one of the Hamar villages near the border of Kenya, a small girl tugs on my hand. She has a scarf slung over her head and wrapped across her body, as if she is hiding behind the tattered red-and-gold fabric. While she looks up at me, a gust of wind blows the scarf away, offering me a full view of her face.

Her left eye is big, bold, brown, framed by leafy lashes. But the other eye is red, severely infected, weepy with green pus.

"Please," she says. "Just one birr." That's the equivalent of four cents.

The Omo Valley is populated by indigenous tribes with rich cultural traditions, like body modification, ritual scarring, body painting, and sacred rites. This is where you'll find the Mursi tribe, where women stretch their lower lips with ornamental plates. Members of the Kara tribe decorate their bodies with elaborate designs using highly pigmented paint made from pulverized minerals mixed with water. Hamar boys are initiated into manhood by running across the backs of fifteen bulls, smeared with dung to make them slippery, at least four times; the Hamar women are voluntarily whipped to demonstrate their support and loyalty to the men.

This area was the crossroads of humanity for thousands of years, where human migration began, and the region is an important link in human evolution, home to significant hominid fossil discoveries. But it is literally and figuratively far removed from the world I know. To get here, it took three long days in a four-wheel-drive vehicle with a guide who knows the tribes, and to pay for it I used the last of my secret stash of U.S. dollars (a stash so secret that I had forgotten about it until I tore apart my backpack looking for something else).

Though the tribes have been established in the valley for hundreds of years, living the same way for centuries, that's changing rapidly. A hydroelectric dam changed the fragile landscape and natural flood cycle of the river. Tribal land has been claimed by the government and leased for commercial farms. Some tribespeople have been forced into resettlement camps.

The area has also seen an increase in tourism, which creates an unsustainable economy and an unnatural power structure between the tribes and visitors. These are dignified people who cannot live the way they have always lived, because they must parade for travelers, and they are discouraged from making progress; these communities cannot make technological advances for risk of losing the influx of tourist dollars. I cannot figure out how to be a responsible visitor here, because my mere presence feels predatory.

I give the child with the infected eye a handful of birr, but I'm not naive enough to think it will help. My spirit is broken. I do not feel determined. I do not feel adventurous. I have traveled to the most remote place I've ever been, and all the world has shown me is more pain.

Someone in the village tells me the girl will be getting attention soon, but I worry it won't be soon enough. Ethiopia has one of the highest rates of blindness in the world. Most of these cases are caused by infectious eye diseases, like the bacterial infection trachoma, and are preventable.

I'm not positive this child has trachoma, but it's so common here that I suspect that's what she has. It spreads quickly through contact with eye discharge, so all it takes is one child wiping their eyes on a mother's skirt or a father's handkerchief, and then the whole village is affected. Poor hygiene facilities—or no facilities at all, which is the case in this village—contribute to the problem, leaving no opportunity to sanitize clothes, wash hands, or clean faces. When I walk away, I scrub my hands with an antibacterial wipe, one of a few I keep in a small first aid kit.

After my encounter with the girl, I visit the local market, where people from the Hamar tribe barter and trade vegetables, livestock, and *tej*, honey wine. The women wear their hair in short locks styled with butter fat and stained with red clay. The men keep their hair closely cropped or their heads shaved. Both men and women have scarred skin from ceremonial cutting and ritual beatings with sticks and thorns. Some of these are beauty marks, but some of the scarification represents success in battle.

Although I am curious about other communities and how they live, which is one of the things I love about travel, I am uncomfortable here, a tourist of people. I can't decide if my presence exploits this culture or helps preserve it. It's only relatively recently that currency was introduced to these tribes, but it overshadows almost all of my interactions. People ask for money in exchange for photos. If I don't want to take photos, they throw rocks until I go away.

The one exception is a matronly woman who approaches me at the market. She wears a skirt of goat hide and fabric, slung loose and low around her hips. She has no shirt, but heavy ropes of cowrie shells and beads swing from her neck.

The woman smiles, takes my hand, and pulls my fingers across the bare skin just under her breasts. I nearly jump back in surprise, not from the ornamental scarring that spirals across her torso like a garland of Braille, but because it's been a long time since I've touched anyone. She urges me to buy some tej, which I do, and we split a bottle. I drink too much, and soon I feel dizzy. We can barely communicate, but she is a scarred woman, and I have scars too.

That night I go to sleep in a shelter with a tin roof and walls made of tree branches and dung. I stay there the whole next day too. There is a rattle in my chest, my head burns with fever, and my stomach is upset. I sleep on the floor and only have enough strength to use the restroom in a bowl on the other side of the room. When a storm passes through, the rain leaks through the roof and leaves sorrowful puddles around me. I cough as though there is something inside me trying to get out.

I am miserable. I've heard that plants are grateful for the cold, and that some flowers only bloom in the mud. The idea is not just that harsh conditions cultivate beautiful things, but also that we have to endure suffering in order to appreciate the lack of suffering. Pain is the necessary element for growth.

I think about the woman at the market and her beautiful, unsettling scars, formed from dozens of tiny cuts. The wounds must have been excruciating until the welts formed, and now they demonstrate how strong she is. But that's the nature of pain, isn't it? You can't cure it; you can't fix it; you only let it heal.

Go to Your Scary Place

Of all the places in the world, India is the only place I don't want to visit, and that's because it sounds daunting. I am intimidated by the things I've seen on the news, which is all I know about India—the country's size, the number of people, the sickness, the depth of poverty. It sounds like too much.

Then Barbara meets up with me in Addis Ababa, where I have returned after the Omo Valley. I'm no longer running a fever, but I'm not well either.

Barbara gives me the used-car-salesman pitch. She says that India is one of those must-see places for every backpacker. She promises it will be transformative.

"You're not a *real* backpacker unless you go to India," she says in an effort to peer-pressure me into it.

It works. Plus I have been spending too much time alone, and I could use the company. Besides, I was the person who talked her into coming to Ethiopia, a place she wasn't exactly keen on seeing. So in an effort to be agreeable, I agree. We arrange visas and purchase tickets, and we will be sitting side by side as we fly into Mumbai, formerly known as Bombay. I'm nervous, but I'm relieved to be exploring a new place with someone familiar.

The night before our flight, Barbara approaches me on the patio at our hostel and says, "Hey. Don't be mad at me, but . . ." Though I don't know exactly what she's going to say, I already know it's going to be bad. Nothing good ever follows that phrase.

There's a guy, she continues.

"And I've decided to go to Berlin with him. My flight leaves in three hours."

It's devastating and disappointing, but I can't even summon the strength to argue. I wish Barbara well, even though I believe she's making a mistake, and I stomp off. I consider veering off course and changing my flight to somewhere that sounds easier to navigate. I could learn to surf in Australia. Go on multi-day hikes in the New Zealand countryside. Explore the beaches of Bali.

But then I wonder if there's some other reason I am bound for India. Maybe this was meant to be. I try to remember if my mom ever said anything about India, and I can't come up with anything. It's possible she was intimidated by the thought of India too.

Kaj, a Canadian journalist I've gotten to know at the hostel bar, sees that I'm upset and buys me a beer. After I spill the story, he writes two bits of advice on a piece of paper. One is the name of an affordable place to stay in Mumbai. The other is the name of a town he's sure I'll love.

I tuck the torn blue paper into my wallet, and it feels more valuable than any of the paper money inside. Faced with a country that feels enormous and strange, having a direction is like finding a treasure map.

I land in Mumbai at 4 a.m. Alone. Exhausted. Frightened and sick. An infection from the grit and pollution of Ethiopia has settled into my lungs, and I can hardly move without sending myself into a coughing fit. My body aches.

I hand over my blue piece of paper to a taxi driver, and we depart in one of Mumbai's iconic yellow-and-black Premier Padmini taxis.

Just past the ring of high-rise hotels that encircle the airport is a sprawling neighborhood of bewildering poverty and neglect. This is Annawadi, one of India's most famous slums, where thousands of people squat on airport property. The sewers are open and flowing. Towers of trash line the maze of roads.

"The first thing I noticed about Bombay was the smell of the different air," writes Gregory David Roberts in the novel *Shantaram*, and that's what hits me as well. The taxi window is down, and the air that rushes into the car is thick, smoky, and bloated with humidity. It smells robust, like perfume and incense, waste and potent spices.

We drive through the slums as dawn breaks. The homes are slim and cramped; life spills out onto the streets. There are people everywhere. Hundreds if not thousands of people beginning work for the day. They carry jugs of water, start fires, brew tea. They pack carts full of fruits and flowers. Neighbors yell to each other. Children wash their faces. Women make food. Dogs bark.

The roads open into a cityscape of stunning architecture, shiny buildings, signs, fabric, stalls, cars, trucks, people, cows. There's a cacophony of horns from all the vehicles that surround us. Every block reveals something beautiful and something strange, and it is everything.

Sure, I have fallen in love with locations at first sight before. Sucre, Bolivia, was one. Another was Sedona, Arizona, during a Christmas road trip with Jason. We arrived at night and couldn't see anything beyond our car's headlights. When we looked out our hotel room in the morning, the sheer beauty of the snow-dusted red mountains felt like a wallop. And now there is Mumbai, which steals my heart immediately with its majesty and color and noise. Being here is like flipping a switch inside; I feel lit from within.

The taxi driver drops me off at the address I requested, a building that looks like every other building in the neighborhood. A white structure grayed by soot and mildew, tangles of electrical wires stretched overhead. When I knock on the door, a grizzled old man opens it, hands me the key to a room, and then shuffles away. He doesn't even ask for payment. I drop my backpack by the bed and head back outside. It takes effort because I'm still struggling to breathe from my lung infection, but Mumbai has already wooed me like a new lover, and I can't imagine staying indoors.

My hotel is within walking distance of the Gateway of India, the enormous basalt arch that proudly stands watch over the Mumbai Harbor, so I catch it in the morning light. A purple spun-sugar mist simmers over the water, and birds fill the air. It is dazzling. Equally dazzling, a man bicycles down the road with trays of eggs stacked on the back in a precarious tower that is taller than he is, a balancing act as beautiful as anything in Cirque du Soleil.

The vendors are just setting up for the day, and I buy a fresh plate of bhel poori, puffed rice tossed with cooked onions and potatoes, drizzled with a tart tamarind sauce, and drink a small mug of chai. It is warm and creamy enough to soothe my prickly throat. Then I visit a pharmacy, where I am given pills and an inhaler for my lungs. I return to my hotel room, take the pills, and sleep for the next two days within the peach-colored walls.

When I wake, my lungs are clear, the cough is nothing more than a scratch in my throat, and my scary place no longer exists. Something has ruptured inside me. This is India, the land of transformation and enchantment, and I'm hungry to experience it.

OVER THE NEXT FEW DAYS, I EXPLORE MUMBAI MOSTLY BY foot. I watch games of cricket, duck into a movie theater to beat the afternoon heat, sip Bombay Sapphire in sleek nightclubs with blue neon lights. I buy looser, flowy clothing, appropriate for the weather, and stuff my hiking pants into the bottom of my backpack. I meet a friend's sister-in-law, Malini, who is in Mumbai on business, and we have a conversation that sinks deep into the night about travel, desire, and what it means to experience life.

Walking past Chhatrapati Shivaji Maharaj Terminus, the magnificent train station formerly known as Victoria Terminus, I'm lured inside by a crush of people. Other travelers have told me that the best way to experience India is by rail, but they warned the act of purchasing tickets can be tricky. I feel lucky when I emerge an hour later with a ticket that night on a sleeper car bound for Goa.

The former Portuguese colony of Goa is known for beaches and laid-back parties. It's where the hippies go. I shamefully didn't do any research about the place—it just sounded far less intimidating than heading north to frenetic New Delhi.

The three people who share the sleeper car with me are also travelers—a British couple and a sweet, baby-faced German named Denis. We become fast friends, and when they disembark at Anjuna Beach, so do I. Denis and I split the last room available at a place called Peace Hostel. We rent scooters, the most efficient way to navigate the congested, palm tree–lined streets, and the best way to cool off when the air is unbearably hot.

Beachy Goa is home to cashew farms, spice plantations, and tropical fruits, so the dishes we eat are laced with coconut milk, nuts, and intense spice blends. Seafood is a staple. And every dish balances the heat of chili peppers with a tart note, either from vinegar (the influence of four centuries as a Portuguese colony) or the native kokum fruit or tamarind. I've eaten Indian food before, but it's never tasted like this, fiery, tangy, and rich at once.

What I love about Denis is that he's young enough to still be excited about the world; he's not jaded in the slightest, and he doesn't carry any hurt yet. We go to parades, tour spice plantations, do yoga, ride the motorbikes to forts and churches, then leave Anjuna and rent a small hut along Palolem Beach. I spend entire afternoons standing in the warm Arabian Sea, water up to my hips, a cold beer bottle in one hand.

In the evenings Denis and I go to crowded bars, people spilling out into the sand. Denis carries around a gallon-sized bag of weed, so he makes friends easily. I don't smoke any of it—it's garbage weed anyway—but I tag along for barefoot walks along the edge of the water. We find fallen palm trees and sit astride them, staring up at the sprinkle of stars overhead, a few stoned people littered about.

Traveling time runs differently than normal time. It doesn't adhere to a strict twenty-four-hour schedule or follow the calendar. Some days unravel in a flash. Some nights are as endless as space. Nobody ever knows the date. Denis has this guiding philosophy—borrowed from a movie he once saw—that while traveling, every day is Saturday. He often shouts it into the screaming wind on the motorbike or howls it at the moon. "Every day is Saturrrdaaaayy!"

One night, maybe Saturday, we attend a silent disco. There's a DJ, but the music can't be heard by anyone in the place unless you're wearing headphones. It's the strangest experience, all of us dancing to the same electronic beat, but separated, something both unifying and isolating.

It's a great metaphor for how I feel traveling through this place. I have made real connections with people. I have friends here, and I haven't been alone in weeks. I'm going through all the motions of a normal backpacker. But I still feel detached from the experience. An invisible fortress of grief surrounds me, and I don't know when those walls will come down. If they ever will. I also know that by walling myself off from grief, I'm also keeping joy at bay.

Before my mom died, I thought sadness was a state that involved tears and melancholy afternoons drowning in music by the Smiths. But sadness can also look like this—sunshine days and party nights, unaware of time itself, digging my feet into the sand just to remind myself I'm still somehow attached to this world. It's a beat nobody else will ever hear.

THE BUS THAT RUMBLES INTO HAMPI HAS TRANSPORTED me to another world—one less crowded than Mumbai, slower even than Anjuna—a land of stately temples, enormous rock formations, and a ruddy red terrain dotted with juicy green fields. It looks like a chunk of India that has been shipped to another planet. This is the second thing written on the piece of paper that Kaj gave me in Ethiopia, and I silently give thanks for his advice. This sacred Hindu holy city is instantly captivating, but it's a tiny dot on a map that I wouldn't have explored otherwise.

My friend Denis has come along, and we've spent the entire ride together in a sleeper car, which is like a tiny cubicle with double beds and a door that slides shut to lock you into place with whatever weirdo is sharing the car. I'm grateful my weirdo is Denis, so the entirety of our trip is spent cracking jokes and mixing cocktails with warm cola and a local alcohol made of cashews. We have so much fun, and none of the other passengers would ever guess it's only been two months since my mom died.

So far I've done my best to shove my grief aside, which is remarkably easy in India since my backpacking friends know me only as Maggie the Traveler. I am the person who will hop on the back of a motorcycle to tour ancient ruins or the person who will stay up late to smoke a hookah and swap stories. They see me as whole because I haven't shown them the broken parts. I am not Maggie the Mourner, I'm not Maggie the Woman with a Dying Mom, and I'm certainly not Maggie Who Has No Mom. These new friends know me and me alone, so far out of the context of my own life, it's like the rest of it never happened. Occasionally I try on other identities, and I figure it's not lying if I'm giving people a good story to tell later. I'm a surfing instructor for dogs. A fortune cookie writer. Geena Davis. I can be anyone I want to be, because the person I least want to be is me.

After procuring a room at a hostel, Denis and I walk up Anjaneya Hill to the Monkey Temple.

The temple is located at the top of 575 steep, bone-white steps that zig-zag up the side of a mountain. When we arrive, monkeys tumble across the rocks, chatter as they hop along the staircase, and climb to the temple roof. I assume that is how Monkey Temple got its name—the actual monkeys that reside here—but it turns out I'm wrong.

This is thought to be the birthplace of Hanuman, represented as a monkey and an incarnation of the Hindu god Shiva. In mythological times, Hanuman was the greatest devotee of Rama, an Indian king. When Rama's brother was wounded, the only cure was an herb that grew only in the Himalayan mountain range—but there was hardly any time. Hanuman is said to have achieved the impossible by leaping from the southern part of India all the way to the Himalayas in the north. When he got there, Hanuman wasn't sure which herb was needed, so he grew to a larger form and carried the entire mountain back with him. Healers were able to pluck the necessary herb, and the life was saved. Hanuman's steadfast devotion and determination have since been lessons for generations of Hindus.

The temple is whitewashed, same as the steps, perched on a plateau like a dollop of whipped cream. A red turret completes the image of a sundae like a cherry on top. The panoramic view of Hampi from this vantage point is breathtaking, with checkerboards of ripe, green fields and rugged, rocky land. Veins of water branch through it.

There is a man with a white beard, a white sheet wrapped around his legs like an oversized diaper, who speaks softly and tells stories about Hanuman. I remove my shoes to enter the holy space, and my feet burn on the hot cobblestones. The man ushers me inside the cool shade of the temple, where I am offered a cup of chai, and I drink it. Then I move through the small space, clockwise. At one of the altars, a Hindu priest presses a finger in a bowl of vermillion powder, then swipes it on my forehead to leave a dot. This is a blessing for my third eye, the place of inner wisdom.

Wisdom hasn't exactly been my strong suit of late, and I feel guilty keeping the dot on my forehead. If anything, I've been purposefully dodging my pain rather than reckoning with it.

I don't think about home much anymore. I don't think at all. I exist in my own numbness, wandering with no real intention, zooming from town to town on motorcycles. I tear through easily digestible novels, like the entire *Pretty Little Liars* series, immersing myself in stories other than my own. I drink and I drink and I drink until I sleep, and when I wake, I drink some more, the epidural to make my discomfort go away.

Somehow I have slipped. I have regressed into the self-destructive, feral person I was in the early days of my mom's illness, and I can't do this anymore. I can't continue pretending I am not hurt as my wounds remain open and sore.

While my mom's journey toward dying made me want to live more vibrantly and fully, it's her death that has caused me to shut down.

Before I leave, the priest pulls me aside and says Hanuman brings peace to agitated minds. My face burns red, as though I've been seen—really seen— for what I am. Maybe he intuited it. Or maybe he knows that everybody struggles with something they hide.

Enlightenment Is Boring

—⦿⦿⦿—

AFTER HAMPI, DENIS AND I HEAD BACK TO GOA, WHERE he's planning on staying for an undetermined amount of time. I know I need to leave, but I don't yet have a destination. We loll on the beach, our sweaty bodies flopped on a sandy blanket, as I try to make a decision.

"Like, everybody needs to go to an ashram," says a nearby woman, who is stupefyingly drunk and wearing a Playboy bikini—and the way she says it makes me think I absolutely do not want to go to an ashram. She makes it sound like a cliché, another box that needs to be ticked off the "Things to Do in India" list, not a place of spiritual retreat and simplicity.

But as time passes, I can't stop thinking about the ashram this woman suggested. After so many nights of mindless drinking and dancing, and too many days of sunning and smoking bidi cigarettes, an ashram sounds like a relief. I need some direction in my life, and it might as well come from someone in a Playboy bikini.

This particular ashram, Sivananda, is snuggled into the hills of southern

India, surrounded by fields and misty mountaintops. The closest neighbor is a lion sanctuary.

By the time I make it there, I am feeling the effects of too much travel and too much grief. My body is bruised, and my head is heavy. Every matriarch in my family is dead. I know I still have a husband and siblings, a father and friends, but I couldn't feel more alone and aimless.

The schedule at Sivananda is rigorous, beginning with meditation at 5 a.m., then continuing with classes, spiritual sessions, and volunteer work throughout the day.

We receive two vegetarian meals per day, served in an expansive dining hall. We file into the room individually and sit on bamboo mats, where we chant before the meal. The food is served on large silver platters with sections, just like in a cafeteria. In addition to no meat or fish, the food is cooked without eggs, garlic, onions, or salt, so every dish is mild. A typical meal is chapati bread, bananas, dal, and a salad with shredded beets, carrots, and cabbage. Volunteers loop around the room and serve up unlimited refills from buckets.

I no longer have any choices to make, which is a relief, since my trip so far has been nothing but one choice after another: Should I stay in Bolivia or go to Argentina? Will I stay two weeks or three? Should I volunteer at the school or the farm? Do I want to stay in the city or in a rural area? Should I take the bus or walk? Should I barter for the fare or not bother?

At the ashram, the constraints are liberating. I am told when to wake up. When to meditate. When to bathe. When to eat. When to do yoga.

And there is so much yoga. Five hours of yoga a day. I am spending more time upside down than I did on my honeymoon.

This yoga is not like any other class I've taken before. First off, there is no sound. No throaty, chanting music. No banging of brass singing bowls. Not even a sitar CD. We also don't flow from one asana to another. We simply move from pose to pose, holding each one for several excruciating minutes at a time. It is not a sweat-it-out workout. It is a physical form of meditation.

After one week, I approach the yoga instructor.

"Hey, I was wondering if we could change the yoga class a little bit," I say. "Mix things up."

"Of course not," he says. "What we're trying to do here is to achieve a higher, more mindful state. Reach enlightenment."

"Okay. It's just kind of boring."

He snaps back, "Enlightenment is boring."

This is the first time I've ever heard those three words in that order, and it's a revelation: enlightenment is boring.

For the past ten years, ever since my mom was diagnosed with Alzheimer's, I've been throwing myself into activities and excursions, assuming adventure was the only way to truly experience life. I've plodded my way around the world; I have literally thrown myself out of perfectly good airplanes. But what if it means this? What if enlightenment is tucked away in the routine of our days?

Maybe I should have been looking for meaning among the mundane all along. It's a sticky thought that stays with me all day and long into the night. I wonder if enlightenment is actually attained in these blank spaces—the long and rambling prairie that grows in between the mountains I've climbed and the oceans I've crossed.

I head back to my dorm, Lakshmi, named for the goddess of prosperity, where I'm one of seventy women. I brush my teeth, scrub my face, and settle onto my flat, hard mattress while turning the questions over in my head. The brassy gong outside signals that it's time for lights-out. My eyes are heavy and then comes an urgent thought, something so swift and powerful that it shakes me wide awake: what if my mom's life was never the boring, unlived journey I presumed it to be?

The night is hot and still, and I lie with that thought for a long time. All this time I've been operating under the assumption that my mom didn't get to accomplish what she wanted to accomplish, simply because she didn't make it to specific destinations. She didn't achieve her goals, or, at least, what I thought her goals were.

But the act of living a life is the act of establishing priorities. Maybe people do what they want to do. And perhaps what my mom wanted to do, more than she wanted the world, was to be with me.

When I realize this, I'm smiling and weeping in the dark.

Like most other women in the dorm, I sleep naked or in my underwear because it's too hot for clothes. Even the most modest among us have shed garments over the past several days, like snakes discarding their old skin. Our unnecessary layers are peeled away. What emerges is fresh and new, revealing.

My only nighttime cover is a thin sarong, brown and pink, threaded with golden fibers, which I bought on the beach in Goa. I pull it over me like a blanket, even though it's as sheer as gauze. It touches me like the lightest kiss. Moisture beads on my skin, and around me, I hear others breathe and moan through their dreams. For the first time since my mom's death, I am not actively grieving. I might even be okay. At some point I fall asleep, though I have no idea how long it is before the night takes me.

The next morning is a special event. Rather than chant in the temple, we are guided through the darkness on a silent, meditative hike. Rocks crunch under my shoes as I make my way, one step at a time, up a slippery trail I can't even see. I am not sleepy, even though I spent hours awake in the dark. If anything, every cell crackles inside my body. I'm as awake as I've ever been.

When we reach the summit, we sit and chant until the sun rises, and when it comes it's almost as though we will it into being. It's a spectacular show, a citrus orange sun drenching the sky with juicy color.

"*Jaya Ganesha!*" my ashram friends sing with jubilance, and several people bang rocks together like cymbals. Far away the lions roar, loud enough to provide bass for our melody. My friend Bhanu strikes a pose on some rocks, and he is like a purple-clad warrior against the vivid sky. When we do yoga, the mountain warms under our palms.

It's possible this is what I've traveled all this way to learn. Enlightenment is boring, and it looks something like this: shuffling through the dark, trusting there's a trail beneath your feet that leads into sunshine, movement, and joy.

FOR THE NEXT COUPLE OF WEEKS, I ZIGZAG AROUND INDIA solo but collecting friends along the way. For two nights I drift on a houseboat in Alleppey with two American backpackers, Jesse and Dave, floating around backwaters and lush canals. I meet a German hiker in Munnar, where the sprawling tea plantations look like rumpled green quilts, and we spend several mornings traveling over verdant hillsides.

But my friends aren't limited to backpackers. In Mysore I am temporarily adopted by a family, and they treat me to a guided tour of the dazzling Mysore Palace, buy me dinner afterward, and then take me to a temple and show me how to pray. They ask for nothing in return, only the opportunity to share this intersection of our lives. In Kolkata I CouchSurf with a twenty-nine-year-old attorney. During my stay he has a party with takeout and close friends to watch the Cricket World Cup semifinals against Pakistan. When India wins, the celebration includes dancing in the streets, banging on buckets like snare drums, and an exhilarating stream of fireworks that glitter against the dark sky.

On a train ride, a Malayali man explains arranged marriages by saying, "In India, love comes after marriage." At first it strikes me as funny, but the more I think about it, the more I can see how that works. Marriages take work, initial attraction fades, and being in love each day is a choice.

It's a strange thing to love Jason and to be so far away from him. I haven't seen him since January, when he met me in Ohio for my mother's funeral, and we have just celebrated our first wedding anniversary on Skype. I sent him a movie and a boxed Indian dinner from Amazon, and then I hunkered in the corner of a restaurant with Wi-Fi and we ate *chana masala* together—two computer screens and 9,000 miles between us. The distance is a strain, though, and so is time, and we are both growing into new people. I once heard someone describe her ex-partner as "the same river but not the same water," and I'm curious if this will be the case when I see Jason again. When two people grow, there's no assurance it will be in the same direction.

I stay for a few nights with a lonely fifty-one-year-old woman in Chennai who lives in an empty house—her children are grown and her husband is often absent, so she opens her home to backpackers and travels vicariously through their stories. She teaches me to cook creamy *dal makhani* out of black lentils, takes me shopping in her favorite markets, and shows me all the tourist sites. She also drives me to the airport when it's time to go. When I say goodbye, she gets out of her car in the parking lot and gathers me into her arms. She instructs me to be safe and to be good. I cry into her shoulder as she cradles me like a mother.

For one of my final days in India, I head to Kanyakumari, the southernmost tip of the country. This is the confluence of three seas—the Bay of Bengal, the Arabian Sea, and the Indian Ocean—and the beaches are multicolored from the different currents that wash crimson, black, and ochre sand ashore from different locations. It's also the holy place where Mahatma Gandhi's ashes were kept in an urn before they were released into the sea.

According to legend, this is where the young goddess Devi Kanyakumari stood, balanced on one foot, praying to be coupled with Lord Shiva. When the marriage was eventually thwarted, the furious and scorned woman cursed the food items that had been prepared for the wedding buffet. In her rage, she tossed the food everywhere, and the rice and grains became the rainbow-hued shore.

I dip my bare feet into the azure waves, water heaving around my ankles, pushing and tugging at my feet, and I feel a confluence of natural forces within me too. Like this intersection of seas, I know I am the result of not one path, but many.

I recall my grandmother, who became a traveler late in her life. She often accompanied a neighbor couple on tours and cruises, then packaged her memories into Kodak slides. When I visited her for my thirteenth birthday, she devoted one entire evening to projecting wonders of the world on her living room wall: the Sphinx, the Taj Mahal, the Acropolis. I slurped grandma's homemade oxtail soup and saw her posed by the Colosseum, both inside and out. The photos were terrible. She either took up the bulk of the frame or was a speck in the distance, and nearly everything seemed to lean—except for the Leaning Tower of Pisa, which was strangely upright.

I don't know what motivated my grandmother to travel, and I won't ever know, but thinking about it now makes me feel close with her in a way I never have before. I wonder in how many places our footprints have overlapped, how the water that licks my feet has touched the shores of places she has been.

It's true for my mom too. There's a chance that this water once bathed her, provided a place to swim, rained on her forehead.

Kanyakumari is a spot where the sun both rises and sets in the water, and while I'm standing there, the ending and beginning that exists in all things flashes inside me. I don't know if I believe in rebirth, but I do believe in hope, and that's almost the same thing. That's the gift I receive here.

My mom no longer lives in this world, but it's only through her passing that I discovered it. This water, this rainbow-littered ground, this sinking sun; it all came to me because of her.

Pave the Way

———∞∞∞———

THE AIR IS MOIST, AND I'M KNEELING ON A HOT SWATH OF road, my baggy cotton fisherman pants sticking to melted bits of pavement, and my T-shirt stuck to the sweatiest parts of my back.

I'm in a rural part of northern Thailand, about an hour-and-a-half drive north of Chiang Mai. There's no semblance of a town in this remote area, just a few scattered roadside cafés and small convenience stores. Nailed to the occasional tree are hand-painted signs advertising treetop zip lines, trekking, or rafting on the nearby Mae Taeng River.

I'm not here for the adrenaline, though. I'm building a road with about ten other people. Together we mix buckets of concrete and smooth over the street's cracks and potholes. In some places, the road is so profoundly crumbled, our patches form the entirety of the street.

It's difficult work, but at least our surroundings are beautiful. There is jungle on each side of the road, a tangle of green, leafy trees, squatty palms, and long, grassy weeds.

This is not what I expected to do when I came here. I signed on to volunteer at an elephant sanctuary because of my mom's love for animals, because she was awed by elephants. She would think the opportunity to care for and be close to gentle giants is a gift. And it is.

Most days I unload truckloads of produce, shovel elephant poop from the shelters, prepare watermelons, bananas, and squash for meals, and help clean the property. The best part of the day is when we lead the elephants to the river for bathing, then goof around and toss buckets of water on each other.

Elephant Nature Park was founded by a woman named Lek; she created the park as a sanctuary and rehabilitation center for elephants that have been injured, abused, or tortured by humans. After elephants were banned from the Thai logging industry in the 1980s, those animals were then forced to work in shows or give rides to people or were used for street begging. So elephants became an essential part of the tourism industry, but they weren't any better off than when they were used for logging. Some are trained with whips, chains, or arrows. Some are given medication to keep them awake through the night for street begging.

Though it's not the most glamorous task, building a road for the sanctuary is another way to help the elephants.

When Lek created the sanctuary and became vocal about the trauma inflicted upon elephants, some government officials were concerned about the repercussions this could have on tourism, and maintenance on the road leading to the sanctuary stopped. That's why I'm filling holes on a sweltering April day. I'm literally paving the way for more volunteers and animal lovers to help elephants.

AFTER THE PATCHWORK ROAD CONSTRUCTION IS COMpleted, my volunteer group is given the afternoon off. We take rubber tubes to the brown expanse of river, where mud clings to the water. We drift through the landscape, through green farmland and rice paddies that run up to the water's edge, through wild jungle, where unruly ferns and fringy palms provide a canopy.

At the start of our trip, we dodge floating lumps of fibrous elephant poop, each about the size and shape of a basketball. (I use a flip-flop to paddle one over in a friend's direction.) But as we continue, the river becomes swift and quick-moving. It runs clear and wide. When we see a village, we bring ourselves to shore. Some people have money tucked into waterproof plastic pouches, and they buy a round of Chang beers in sweaty glass bottles for everyone.

That night is one of my last in the Elephant Nature Park, although I would be content staying much longer. I've done what I've come here to do, which is slow down, spend time in nature, tend to something bigger than myself. I feel like I've made a contribution.

My mom would be proud of this, I think.

There are two elephants I wish I could tell her about, Mae Perm and Jokia, who have been best friends for years.

Mae Perm worked in logging until the ban in 1989, then was kept as a pet with a poor diet and numerous health problems. When her owners decided to sell her in 1992, she became one of Lek's first rescues. Jokia, who was also abused as a logging elephant, arrived at the sanctuary in 1999. While she was pregnant and working in the logging industry, she gave birth in the jungle to a calf, who rolled down a hill and perished. Jokia was beaten to continue her work, and when she refused, her mahout shot her with a slingshot and blinded her in one eye. With her continued refusal to work with the logs, the mahout attempted to break her. When he stabbed her in the other eye, he left her completely blind.

The two rescues became fast friends at the park, where Mae Perm made herself into Jokia's constant companion and refused to leave her side. She leads Jokia through the park, trundling forward, with a mighty trunk that reaches out to offer the occasional tender pat, and reassures her with a low rumbly sound.

It's fascinating and moving and comforting to realize the most massive animals have the strongest hearts. I've heard before that elephants demonstrate grief for their own, but now I've seen firsthand how the elephants show tenderness and nurture one another. The relationship between Mae Perm and Jokia feels both maternal and old, as though the most basic instinct is for these two animals to tend to each other.

Beyond the elephants, I have one additional creature I tend to during my stay. Stick Dog is a yellow mutt with short fur and joints that have been rubbed raw and pink from sleeping on the ground. His ears are two little triangles that point right up to the sky, and his tongue is dappled with gray spots. He always, always carries the same stick, a broken branch about a foot long, as thick as a hoagie.

Stick Dog began following me around the day I arrived. After two days he started to sleep at the door of my bungalow. If I hadn't been sharing the room with two other women, I would have let him inside.

He carries the stick even as he clambers up the rickety wooden stairs to the bungalow. Then he curls himself up carefully, still with the stick situated in his mouth. Since he's become a frequent visitor, I put a blue plastic bowl of water outside my door and sneak a little extra food from the lunch line. Only then does Stick Dog put the stick down, and only for a brief pause before he snatches it up again.

"What's the deal with the stick?" I ask one of the full-time staff members.

Like most of the animals at the elephant sanctuary, the story of Stick Dog is another of trauma and resilience. Stick Dog's previous owner was quick to beat the dog with whatever happened to be lying around; in most cases, that happened to be a stick. He came to the park frightened and skinny, his skin exposed and raw with open wounds that he licked until they became infected.

After Stick Dog was rescued by the sanctuary—the story of how exactly that happened is a little unclear—the dog gained confidence. He became assured. He carried his own stick, and he was never without it; nobody was going to hurt him again.

Stick Dog is an example of the anguish that the powerful can inflict upon the weak. Even the elephants are an example of that. But they also show extreme fortitude—how living things can rebound from suffering, how wounds close, how life after pain can be a renewal.

The dusk that settles in this part of the world is purple and misty from the humidity. There is a spider looping a web around the railing that surrounds the bungalow patio. Stick Dog lies against my legs, which are imperfect and marked with hot mosquito bites. For one moment, the dog puts the stick down and allows me to take his muzzle in my hands. I give him a long, hard scritch on the nose, and his tail thumps with pleasure. He is a good boy.

FINISHED WITH MY VOLUNTEER WORK, I RETURN TO THE city of Chiang Mai in time for Songkran, the Thai New Year celebration and water festival. The ancient festival is a time of movement, a passage, when an old year becomes a new one. During Songkran, everything is made fresh.

The traditions originated with cleansing rituals—visiting Buddhist temples and monasteries to sprinkle water over the Buddha statues, pour water over the monks, and say prayers in honor of fresh beginnings.

Over time, this evolved into a massive water fight, involving everyone in the community. Yes, a water fight. The kind with squirt guns and water balloons. In most parts of Thailand, the celebration runs from April 13 to 15, but in Chiang Mai, the party doesn't stop for six days.

The fact that I bought a thin plastic poncho at the beginning of the festival shows both my ignorance and my naiveté. The moment I walk outside my hostel doors, I am wet. Truckloads of people drive down the streets, equipped with barrels and buckets, shoveling water as though they are bailing out a sinking boat. Some people have rigged up hoses by the moat that surrounds the city, and everybody who walks past is sprayed with mossy green water, including me.

A plump monk races down the street toward me, packing a massive, assault weapon–style water gun, and his saffron robe clings to him like apricot glaze on a pork chop. I just barely escape, ducking into a 7-Eleven to catch my breath. I'm wearing the plastic poncho, but I know already it's a pointless act. It's been less than ten minutes since I left my hostel, and my T-shirt and pants are soaked. I grab some junk food and a can of beer to take back to my room. But when I stand in front of the cashier to pay, he pulls a tiny water pistol from beneath the counter and shoots me in the face. Then he warmly wishes me a happy New Year, a new start.

Time Is the Destroyer of All Things

———— ✻✻✻ ————

MY FRIEND ANGIE FROM HOME MEETS ME IN BANGKOK, where she treats me to a nice hotel room with all the amenities—a pool, air conditioning, a mattress with springs. But after a few days of sightseeing, we are headed for another country.

I feel obliged to show Angie a terrific time, as this is her first time in Asia, and I'm nervous about taking her overland to Cambodia. For one thing, there's an ongoing conflict at the border, though all of the violence has been north of our destination, Poipet. Also other backpackers have told me the border crossing is notoriously shady, and even the most experienced travelers are scammed out of their money.

The problems begin almost immediately. The cab driver who is supposed to take us to the bus station refuses to use a meter. He only wants to charge a flat fee, which I know is too hefty. When I insist on a meter, he stops the cab and throws us out.

We eventually get to the bus station. At this point I've been backpacking long enough that I know to look at the bus before I buy a ticket. The bus to Poipet is nice, with plush seats, air conditioning, and TVs that will show movies during the five-hour ride, so Angie and I make the purchase. What I don't expect is this: an hour into the trip, the driver pulls the bus over on a rural road, and all of us passengers are transferred to a rickety bus with no air conditioning, broken windows, and hard, plastic seats.

The highlight of the ride is that there's a small Cambodian girl, about two years old, sitting with her mother in front of me. She peers through the crack in the seat, curious. I smile. She giggles and turns away. Moments later, she turns toward me again, but I duck my head beneath the seat. This game of peekaboo continues for a long time through the Thai countryside. When the girl finally tires and settles into her mother's side for a nap, there's a sad, heavy pain in my chest. I think I'd like a child to find that kind of comfort and shelter in me.

When the bus stops hours later, Angie and I still haven't reached our destination. In order to get to the border, where we can catch a bus on the other side, we need a rickshaw to take us another seven kilometers.

Instead of the border, our rickshaw driver brings us to an office that looks more like a diner.

"Maggie, I don't like this," Angie says, and I don't like it either. But I try to assume control of the situation. I feel like I should have known better, like I should have been able to avoid being taken for a literal ride, but I don't know what I could have done differently.

I refuse to get out of the vehicle and tell the driver to take us to the real border crossing. The driver nods and says he will take us to the *real* place for our Thai exit stamp. We putter down the road a little more, passing small homes and cows, roadside shops and vendors pushing handcarts. We come to a halt in front of a building with a cardboard sign that says "VISA BOARDER," with magazine cutouts like a ransom letter.

Angie and I both shake our heads. No.

At last the driver takes us to a huge gated building with official-looking seals on it. This building looks more like an embassy than anything we've seen yet, until we step inside. There are no desks, no queues, no computers. Just two old men playing chess. One man says the twenty-dollar Cambodian visa will be fifty dollars. I refuse to pay.

Incredibly, the *tuk-tuk* driver is still outside, waiting for Angie and me. I tell him this is his last chance. Either take us to the border, or we won't pay him. I don't know if this makes me an ugly tourist or a smart one, but I am tired.

At the real border, the process moves smoothly. I receive my Thai exit stamp and the twenty-dollar Cambodian visa. Then a policeman examines the passports and gives Angie and me two choices: we can either retrieve the passports from him the following day or pay three dollars now for "express service." My wallet is almost empty, but I can't hand him the money fast enough.

We cross the border on foot, underneath an archway that looks like the putt-putt golf version of Angkor Wat, and then a shuttle takes all the tourists to a transportation center where our options are certainly overpriced. We don't care anymore. Angie and I have been traveling for more than eight hours, and we still have at least two more to go before we even get close to the home where we'll be staying in Siem Reap.

We hire a cab, who drops us off on the outskirts of town and arranges a free rickshaw ride that isn't really free; the rickshaw driver drops us off at a café and demands payment, I'm out of cash, and when I call the friend who is supposed to be giving us a place to stay, her phone is busy. Then I'm crying in a café. I've let Angie down; I've let everybody down. I'm tired of movement. I want to stop. Make it stop.

Angie buys me a can of beer. She puts an arm around me and doesn't say anything, because a good friend doesn't have to. We sit and let Siem Reap bustle around us, with twinkling fairy lights, shoppers and caftan vendors and drunk tourists, men pushing carts full of pineapples and women in silky smocks offering foot massages, shops advertising ice cream and cocktails and baguettes, and in that moment, our stillness feels like an act of rebellion.

I don't know how much time passes before a phone call goes through to my friend Jill, who shows up in a car. She swoops us up, brings us to her house, and tucks us into bed. From that moment on, Cambodia is a relief.

I MET JILL AND HER HUSBAND, BILL, IN PALM SPRINGS. The couple are adventurers by nature and have traveled all over the globe, leading tours through China, Thailand, Peru, Israel, New Zealand, and even Mount Everest base camp. When they traveled to Cambodia, though, they had no idea how much their lives would change.

Bill had heard stories about Aki Ra, a former child soldier who once placed landmines for the Khmer Rouge. As an adult, Aki Ra wanted to make amends for the past, so he sought out landmines with a stick and deactivated the explosives by hand, created a museum to teach visitors about the horrors of landmines, and opened a facility to care for dozens of children who had been wounded by landmines. (Though the conflict has long ended and it's impossible to know how many explosives remain active in Cambodia, an estimated 6 to 10 million still pepper the jungles, fields, and farmland. The weapons continue to maim or kill thousands of children, farmers, and other civilians every year.)

During his first visit to Siem Reap, Bill found Aki Ra and was impressed by the man. Here was someone willing to place his life on the line to better his community and elevate the lives of his neighbors. He was someone focused on making the future better, not dwelling on the past.

Bill, who has eleven marathons under his belt and has climbed Mount Kilimanjaro, is someone who knows how to get things done. He sold his marketing consulting business in Palm Springs and then assisted Aki Ra with getting the proper certification and equipment to legally and safely remove the mines. He learned everything there was to know about finding explosives and disarming them, and he came up with a plan to train and employ Cambodian teams of deminers. Then he established a nonprofit organization, the Landmine Relief Fund, to pay for these efforts.

Finally Bill and Jill packed up their belongings, sold their house, and moved to Cambodia for the rest of their lives. While most people settled down for their retirement years, Bill and Jill reinvented themselves. The great thing about having friends who do selfless work is that their actions inspire me just by bearing witness. The bad thing is that it makes me question if I'm doing enough with my own life.

It's easy to see why Cambodia carved a place in their hearts. There are pink lotus blossoms, pale like a tinted lip gloss, that float over glassy ponds. There are monkeys that tumble alongside the red-orange dirt roads. And of course the temples are remarkable, among the largest religious structures on earth and an artistic achievement.

STANDING BEFORE ANGKOR WAT, I SEE THE TEMPLE NOT just through my own eyes, but also slightly disassociated from my body.

I remember the copy of *National Geographic* in which I saw Angkor for the first time. I was maybe six or seven, and the cover image floored me. It was simply a carved stone face with cracks, bisected by a green vine that promised new life. The headline to the right of the carving said, "The Temples of Angkor: Will They Survive?"

At that time, Cambodia was the Coalition Government of Democratic Kampuchea, and the temple complex was controlled by government troops. Hardly anyone had seen the temples since the Khmer Rouge took control of the nation. Some thought the structures had been severely damaged or demolished—until a *National Geographic* writer, editor, and photographer were granted entry to see the seventy-two major monuments. What they catalogued for the magazine was an architectural wonder of the world that had been damaged by war, conflict, vandalism, and the surrounding jungle, but it still existed, was still magnificent, and was not beyond the point of preservation.

The articles were accompanied by maps, aerial images, illustrations, and close-ups of bas-reliefs, each page more enchanting than the next. I had never seen anything like it, and my mother hadn't either. I remember the wistful tone in her voice, the cock of her head, the way she tucked a blonde curl of hair behind her ear. This was a place she desired to go, but in the 1980s, it seemed unlikely. Angkor was about as attainable as Atlantis.

Now I'm here. The temple that looms before me is not in a magazine. I see the majestic spires, the elegant bas-relief carvings, the expansive complex that is probably bigger than my hometown. The five peaks of the central building are supposed to symbolize Mount Meru, a sacred golden mountain that is considered by some religions to be the center of the universe and to exist in both spiritual and physical planes. The way the sunlight hits this tower now, I can envision it—as though I'm standing in that mythical place and only my feet are still on a ruddy dirt path in the jungle.

I see all this with my own eyes, but I also absorb it through the lens of my mom as well. This is awesome in the purest sense of the word.

The Siem Reap province contains dozens of Buddhist and Hindu temples, most of which date back to the twelfth century. It's a UNESCO World Heritage Site, which means that people flock to the archeological park from all over the globe, but none of them are as excited as me. They can't be.

I am comforted by these ancient spaces. I do think about all the now-dead people who have passed through the same doorways and passages where I walk now, but more than that, I think about the life that existed here. How many people loved and danced, prayed and cried, took vows, made jokes, sang songs, chanted long into the night? How many mothers have held their daughters' hands? How many people mourned? How many people were just like me—carrying around three months of fresh grief, or ten years and three months of extended grief, struggling under the weight of emotional baggage?

Those people might have been lost to memory, but I know that matter stays here on earth. We are made of tiny particles, and it relieves me to think that the smallest pieces of people remain here, that atoms of all walks of life exist here—some of them strangers to me but possibly some of them relatives too. They have mingled with the ground and the air, they have become part of this silent city itself, and I stand with them and among them and breathe them in.

My family doesn't have a mythology to call its own, but here, in a vast temple that has seen layer upon layer of life, I believe I am a part of an intricate and special network.

Later I walk around a relatively small tenth-century temple called Banteay Srei, which instantly becomes my favorite. Compared to Angkor Wat, this temple feels tiny, like a music box, but the carvings are even more intricate and spectacular. It's constructed out of pink sandstone, and some of the bas-relief panels have been deepened with moss and the shadows of centuries. The temple was dedicated to the Hindu deity Shiva, and most of the carvings are feminine with decorative borders; leafy, ornamental swirls; fantastical birds; and beautiful women. There's one woman in particular who resembles my mother in her strong nose, the spread of her hips, the slight smile of her lips. The figure is an *apsara*, a supernatural female spirit of the clouds and waters, and with one hand up by her shoulder, the other extended, it looks like she is poised to ask someone to dance. Seeing her is like looking at someone I know, but slightly rearranged, like looking at a loved one in a dream.

Looming over the entire scene is a carving of Kala, a mischievous-looking character who represents time, the destroyer of all things.

AFTER SIEM REAP, ANGIE AND I SPEND SEVERAL DAYS EXploring the busy capital city of Phnom Penh. The city feels sprawling and cosmopolitan. We take a boat trip along the "four faces"—the place where the Mekong and Tonle Sap rivers meet the lower Mekong and Bassac rivers. We get massages and have cocktails at the Foreign Correspondents' Club along the waterfront. We take a Khmer cooking class. We pay our respects to the dead at the Tuol Sleng Genocide Museum.

During one last excursion before Angie heads home, we make a shopping trip to the Tuol Tompoung in Phnom Penh, more often known as the Russian Market for its popularity among Russian shoppers and expatriates. It's lively and confusing, a maze of vendors selling everything from fine textiles and silver jewelry to (probably fake) Rolex watches and whiskey bottles with dead cobras coiled inside. There are tables piled with brand-name clothing, like Banana Republic and J.Crew—items that are made in Cambodia and sold at steep discounts here—as well as high-end handbags at bargain prices. Also piles of sunglasses. Everybody loves Ray-Bans.

The stalls are pinched closely together, covered by a patchwork of corrugated metal and colorful cloth awnings, filtering the hot, late-afternoon sun into beams of blue and pink light. The overlapping umbrellas of cafés form a ring around the market, where sweaty and hardworking cooks dunk noodles into hot metal pots of soup, grill meat on sticks, and artfully chop up bags of fruit. Plastic chairs and tables overflow into the chaotic streets, where even more shops and restaurants line the roads.

I'm in the market when I see a Western man. He's older, standing stiffly in an intersection of stalls, where a rainbow of embroidered cloth purses hang all the way to the ceiling and baseball caps are sold alongside alleged antiquities. The man appears overwhelmed, like most every tourist here, but there's something else. It's a familiar look in his eyes. I know it. I've seen it a million times in my mother's.

I'm not a doctor, so I can't diagnose him. I don't know if he has Alzheimer's or some other type of dementia. But his gaze is empty, as though he's trying make sense of a 3D image with a hidden picture inside. I am certain he is lost.

I approach him gently and touch him on the shoulder.

"Can I help you find something?" I say.

A wave of relief crashes over his face, and his words tumble out, tripping over themselves, not forming a full sentence: "I'm just … my driver … I don't know where … I can't … my hotel?" and finally he says he can't find his way outside.

I introduce myself, and I take the tall, rumpled man by the arm. I'm happy to show him the way, I say, even though I'm not sure if I should be taking this on. What happens once we get outside? Am I responsible for him? But I know I would feel guilty leaving him inside the market, disoriented and alone.

There were people who did this for my mom. They counted her money at the grocery store, located her car in a busy parking lot, and helped her find her way home again. Maybe some people took advantage of her too; I'll never know. One thing that will always haunt me is the fact that my mom was still involved in the world for a long time before my family realized she needed some protection from it.

This man and I walk through the labyrinthian hallways toward the main entrance, which seems like the most likely place to go. I have my arm looped through his, like he's my genteel grandfather, and occasionally I have to tug at the man to keep him moving in the right direction, not wandering into a stall. Along the way I ask for his name, and he doesn't know it.

What he does remember are Catholic saints, and he tells me that I'm like St. Anthony, a thirteenth-century Franciscan priest, the finder of lost things.

"I used to ask St. Anthony to find my car keys," the man says, grinning. "Now I'm always asking him to find myself."

We chat a little more about patron saints—I briefly attended Our Lady of the Rosary for elementary school, and sometimes I surprise myself by plucking random Catholic factoids out of my brain like a bear snatching a fish from a fast-moving stream—and then we arrive at the entrance of the market.

"Martin!" a Cambodian man shouts.

The man at my side looks across a buzzy crush of people, and the light snaps into his eyes again.

"That's me!" he says. "I'm Martin."

The eagerly waving Cambodian man is his driver. I guide Martin across the street to the place where the man is waiting next to a tuk-tuk. There is a nice leather messenger bag on the backseat and an open soda can on the floor. When I talk to the driver, it's clear the two are well-acquainted; the driver says he has been taking care of Martin for a few days around Phnom Penh. Usually he accompanies Martin, but for some reason today Martin wanted to venture into the market by himself. He had been in there for hours; at this point, the driver wasn't sure if he should go look for the man or stay with the vehicle, where the two agreed they would meet up again.

From what I can tell from this brief conversation, Martin made this trip from the United States to Cambodia by himself. I don't know why, and I'm not sure how long he's been traveling or where he intends to go. I only know he's been relying on the goodwill of others to help him stay the course.

People with Alzheimer's or other types of dementia often experience "sundowning," when they become agitated and confused late in the day and into the night. They wander. They pace. They are restless. Maybe traveling to Cambodia was Martin's version of sundowning, a restlessness that involved changing continents.

My family expected my mom to wander when she still lived at home, which is why we put stop signs on the door and outfitted her with a GPS-tracking-device wristwatch, but she never went far. What she did was prowl the downstairs of the house, shuffling from one room to the next, wringing her hands, as though she had forgotten something. It was always something just out of reach, like trying to retrieve a dream that had already dissipated, the memory evanescent. Whenever we encouraged her to sit or to rest, it only made her irritable and aggressive, so we let her pace until it was time for bed.

Often she looked out the window at passing cars. Sometimes she stared at the Hummel figurines and glass animals in the china cabinet, treasures she put on layaway and obtained one by one; by the time she was diagnosed with Alzheimer's, she didn't remember them at all. They were things that gathered dust.

I recall trying to settle my mom one night. She stood by the living room window, her back to me, angry because I told her she needed to get some sleep. When she finally turned to face me, she swung around so fast, I thought she was going to strike me, which was unlike her but typical of a confused and frustrated person with Alzheimer's.

Instead she wobbled for a minute and then steadied herself. She looked vulnerable, a face crumpled with exhaustion, a woman who had been wrestling with demons. She touched a hand to her forehead, then pressed down on her temple.

"My head. Why does it hurt?"

Let Go

I AM WAIST-DEEP IN BRASSIERES.

The shopkeeper thrusts more and more lacy lingerie my way while pulling from a Jenga tower of ribbons, tulle, and silk that threatens to engulf us both. I know this was probably a mistake—the market in Hanoi would be a better choice for picking up new luggage or an umbrella—but I need a new bra, and right now this market is the best option I have.

I've been traveling for eleven months now with the same two bras. They are utilitarian. One is black, one is nude, neither is pretty. Over time, they have both started to fall apart, but the nude one has sustained considerably more damage. It was stained a weird gray after sharing the wash with Thai pants that leaked blue dye. It smells like a musty gym sock, thanks to a Laundromat that stuffed my washed clothes into a plastic bag before they were dry. I no longer want this bra close to my skin.

The piles of pretty lace at the market are seductive, and I want those new, frilly things. They look so feminine and joyful and clean. I want to be that clean. I want clothes that are frivolous and impractical, underthings with bows, something that will chafe if I wear it on a hike. But today, I will settle for a bra that fits. Any bra. And this is proving to be a challenge.

The shopkeeper doesn't speak English (because why would she?) and I don't speak Vietnamese.

She hands me bras that look like wispy handkerchiefs, bras so flat they are practically concave, and push-up bras with something that feels like raw chicken positioned in each cup.

I try to communicate that I need something more substantial. I point to my chest. I cup my hands in front of my body and make a sinking gesture with my palms. "Big," I say. "Very large."

The woman nods. She pulls out more bras. She tosses them in my direction, rapid-fire, like a blackjack dealer.

Some of them are horrifically ugly with rhinestoned florals, garish crimson with gold sequins, cartoon characters. But most of them simply have no chance of fitting around my frame. It makes me think back to Buenos Aires and all the jeans I attempted to squeeze my body into. Back then, I thought the problem resided with my body; I was trying to conform to another canister, to shape my body into something that wasn't mine. Now I see that my body is fine. It's the clothes that don't work.

I point to my chest again, and inexplicably I sound like the Incredible Hulk at a fruit stand. "Need big," I say. "Big like mango."

By now a small crowd has formed. They have come from the perfume stalls, the shoe stalls, the purse stalls. They gape at me, and I should be self-conscious, but I'm not. I recognize how bizarre I must look, a frazzled white woman hoisting her own breasts in the air, hollering, "Bigger!"

The shopkeeper nods. We go through the whole thing again. More bras, none that will ever fit because all of them have tags that say "A." I point to the tag and scribble down letters. "C"? "D"? Heck, "Z"?

The shopkeeper plunges into the recesses of her stall, and I wait.

I think of my mom all the time, of course, but the memories are strongest when I'm shopping for clothes. My mom loved pretty things. She loved slipping into something new, becoming a different person. We didn't have much money, but she always dressed well. She often put clothes on layaway, paying them off a little at a time, until she could slide them into her closet. She stain-treated items carefully, washed them lovingly—by hand, if she had to—line dried in the backyard, pressed with an iron and spray starch, and then hung them in her closet again. When her closet got too full, my dad bought a separate wardrobe for her dresses, blouses, and sweaters. She loved to buy clothes for me too, even though our tastes didn't match so our choice in clothes rarely did.

The first time she brought me bra shopping, it was because I was required to wear a uniform at Our Lady of the Rosary. The Peter Pan collar shirt I had to wear each day, my choice of white or light blue, was made out of thin fabric, and I was self-conscious about my budding body. I began to wear undershirts to put one more layer between my body and the world. I don't remember which boy noticed, but someone named Jeremy or Brian or Brad saw the strap and assumed it was a bra. Then that kid spread the word that I was the sluttiest girl in our fourth-grade class because I wore a bra and none of the other girls did. (His logic was flawed, but so is the logic of many fourth-grade boys.) Soon afterward, I asked my mom to take me bra shopping, and she was surprised, but I wanted to own that. If I was going to be shamed by my class, at least let me claim the source of it.

Those first bras were white and pale pink with tiny rosettes sewn into the front strap at the base of the two cups (and I use the term "cups" loosely, because that's how they hung on me). They were delicate, but I wasn't. That boy at my school intended to insult me, to steal my power. But even at that young age I knew clothing could act as armor, even the pieces that hid under a uniform. I felt mightier when I had them on.

The Vietnamese shopkeeper emerges, one bra in hand, and a look of calm washes over her face. She plops down a pretty white lace bra with cups as big and round as soup bowls. She nudges it my way and says, "Try."

So I try. There is no dressing room, so I stretch the bra on top of my brown dress. I swear every woman in the circle around me is holding her breath—they're invested in this too. I strike a pose and model it for the crowd. They clap. Success!

Next comes the part where we haggle over the price. However, after rummaging through hundreds of bras and finding only one that fits, there is little room for negotiation. I want that bra, and the shopkeeper knows it. She asks for the equivalent of seven dollars, and I pay it, happily.

THE BRA WAS THE FINAL ITEM I HAD TO PACK BEFORE LEAV-ing Hanoi and continuing on to the next part of my journey. I hoist my backpack onto my shoulders, then catch a ride on a scooter that zips through the congested and lively streets of frenetic Hanoi. The driver drops me off at a travel company storefront, where a bus is waiting to take me to my next destination. And it's an emotional one.

I know of the bay only from photos, but the place in those images looks dramatic, mystical, dreamy. Like nothing else I've seen before on earth. The water is either emerald green, turquoise, or sapphire blue, depending on the light and time of day. Clusters of craggy gray limestone formations rise from the bay like mythical creatures. It's fitting, since "Ha Long" in Vietnamese means "descending dragon."

Legend has it that centuries ago, the newly formed country of Vietnam faced fierce invaders who approached by sea. In retaliation, the jade emperor, who served as the king of heaven, sent a mother dragon and her children to earth to help Vietnam's people defend their country. When the mighty mother dragon and her babies appeared, they breathed fire and spat out pieces of jade the size of mountains, forming a barrier that the battleships couldn't navigate. The enemies who couldn't maneuver around the walls were destroyed; the rest retreated. Over time, the massive jade chunks turned into 1,600 islands of different shapes and sizes, giving us the Ha Long Bay we see today.

When I began this backpacking trip, I told myself it would be a success if I just made it to Ha Long Bay. It was a mental thing, the part of this journey I had to complete. On some of my roughest days, Ha Long Bay was my carrot at the end of a stick; to keep going I looked at images of misty islands among emerald-tinted water.

I don't know what sparked this desire. My mom never dreamt of Vietnam. It was not a place she wanted to go. Because my dad served in the air force in Vietnam, it was only the backdrop of war and conflict for her. It was the place that took her husband for a year, the reason he was away from his children, the reason she received letters instead of his touch.

But I don't carry any of that. My dad never talked about his time in Vietnam, and my history classes at school never managed to make it to the Vietnam War era, so I have nothing to imprint upon this country. Nothing but postcard fantasy images of farmers in conical hats walking through terraces of rice paddies in the Sapa countryside, the colorful merchant houses that line old town Hoi An, and spellbinding Ha Long Bay.

The bus arrives, and it brings me to my home for the weekend, a wooden junk ship with broad, brick-colored sails. They look like scalloped shells cupping the modest breeze. The ship is three levels high with a sundeck on top. My cabin is located along the main deck. After I drop my luggage inside the cabin and open my door again, it looks as though I could step directly onto the water if not for a slender, polished wood railing.

The weather is sunny and calm, the water placid and clear enough that I see multitudes of fish swimming beside the boat as we skim through the bay. Our day involves a trip to Sung Sot grotto, which means surprise grotto, an impressive cavern that was rediscovered by the French in the early 1900s; kayaking around the islands, past pearl farms and homes on stilts; and a dinner cruise at sunset. The captain of this ship maneuvers our boat into a spot that seems to be far away from other cruise ships, but after he sets anchor, more boats gather around us. And then we have a karaoke party.

When I imagined myself in Ha Long Bay, I didn't expect I'd be drinking watery Saigon Special beer and belting out Bon Jovi on a tinny mic. But that's what I got, and I am not disappointed in the least.

We never experience the world exactly as it is. We bring our expectations to a moment, and then we see that through varying lenses of hope, grief, and disappointment—especially the despair that descends when something doesn't live up to the idea we have constructed. That's why it's difficult for travel to meet expectations, and why places don't live up to the hype. They can't. We spend our lives chasing the excitement of the new and the flutter of anticipation, but travel means reckoning with real life.

I think if I came to Ha Long Bay as the same traveler who started my trip just under a year ago, I would have been disappointed by the more commercial, touristy aspects. But what I'm learning is that making memories involves accepting the world the way it comes to you, not the way you wish it to be. It's bellowing "Livin' on a Prayer" under kitschy rainbow-colored lights while floating through one of the most exquisite natural landscapes on earth. It's meeting a place as is.

In the morning, I wake before almost anyone else on the junk. Everything is quiet. I open the cabin door, and I am greeted by a misty green morning. The fog slithers around the limestone rocks, jagged tops peeking over the clouds. I am so close to the water, but the smell here is not briny or fishy; it's more like wet garden. The air is chilly enough that I pull a sarong over my shoulders, but anything else would be too heavy as the sun rises gentle gold and abundant.

My mom didn't know enough about Vietnam to have wanted this, but she would have been enchanted by the juxtaposition of the ragged stone and glass-like water, the calmness that settles with the early morning mist, the ghosts of dragons.

Seeing Ha Long Bay at sunrise is like discovering the key that opens my lock. I stand here for a long time feeling the full weight of this moment and the ease of it too.

If I accept the world as is, that means me too. The bay is still, I feel alone in it, and I am not lonely.

In this instant, I am grateful; I'm practically spilling over. When my mom was diagnosed with Alzheimer's disease, I thought my world was ending. Instead it was just cracking open, finding a way to let something else inside.

There was a time when I thought the world wasn't available to me. My lot in life was that I was from small-town Ohio, and that's where I would stay, even though I desperately wanted to leave. I didn't think I had the skills necessary to do anything else; I didn't think I was capable of following through on my dreams. Now I can't imagine going back to that emotional place ever again. I have been shaken loose, propelled forward, inspired.

The foggy morning gives way to a brilliant afternoon. I spend it with my new friends from the boat. We sprawl out on the sundeck, and when it gets too warm, everyone begins to cannonball into the water, three stories below. Everyone but me.

I stand on top of the railing, one hand clinging to a pole alongside the boat. Everyone below is smiling and laughing, urging me to jump, but I'm frightened. Yes, I have jumped out of airplanes. But when you're looking out of a plane, nothing is relative, so the height barely registers. Here I am fully aware of how high I am and how far I have to fall.

"Do it," yells a woman from Ireland. "Let go."

I screw my eyes shut, take a deep breath, and loosen my grip. Before I even have time to be frightened, I am plunged into the deep and bob to the surface again. I had braced for the hit of cold water, but the bay is bathtub warm, like an embrace. Around me the gentle waves seem to sparkle with glitter as they shift in the sunlight. The protruding rock islands are a vivid shamrock color, the sky a deep teal. Treading water, I am no longer looking at Ha Long Bay or absorbing it from a distance, I am a part of it.

Loving my mom through Alzheimer's was like ten years of digging a tunnel with a spoon, only to discover that the hole I made was a grave. But if my family was going to have that trauma anyway, if we were going to have to dig that grave alongside her, at least I have discovered the magical place on the other side of it all.

My mother deliberately brought me into this world, and I can finally say I've made good on that deal. I am here. I am alive. I am floating in Ha Long Bay, a place that unfolds generously green and merciful, waiting for me to jump so it can show me how buoyant I am.

Look for the Flowers

WHEN I THINK ABOUT MY MOM NOW, THERE ARE ALMOST always flowers: the lily of the valley soap she treasured from Germany, the marigolds and geraniums she planted in the flower boxes of our front yard, the intoxicating purple hyacinth she bought every Easter. Her clothes were dotted with blooms, and when it came time to choose art to hang above our living room couch, she picked out an oil painting with splashy red poppies. In one of my first memories, I'm toddling around our overgrown backyard, where morning glories and tall grasses wove through the chain-link fence like vibrant yarn on a loom; my mom plucks a honeysuckle blossom and holds it to my fat, eager tongue so I can drink the syrupy nectar.

It seems strange then that my mom was buried in a frozen, flowerless landscape. Perhaps there were flower arrangements at her funeral service—that seems probable—but if there were, I don't remember them.

What we did have was a bare, gnarled tree branch, about the length of my arm, which I stuck inside of a vase at the funeral home. I left paper tags on the table next to the vase and asked guests to write their memories of my mom and hang them from the branch.

My family thought it was a silly thing, and as I was trying to make the display perfect, someone pulled me aside to say, "It's okay if you don't have the tree branch. You don't have to do this." I insisted.

I can't articulate why it was so important for me to create that tree branch of remembered moments. Maybe I wanted to know that my mom's life mattered to someone other than me, and the paper tags were a tangible representation. Maybe I simply wanted to take all these memories of my mother and hold them for myself. Maybe I just wanted to watch as the rootless, broken branch—plucked from my parents' backyard on an ashen afternoon—flourished into something beautiful.

As the visiting hours progressed, the bare, naked branch became a blooming thing, each stick coming alive with origami-like blossoms, shivering. It was proof that even in a world without my mom, things could still thrive.

It's been four months since my mom was buried, and I'm a long way from where she rests. I'm headed toward a jungle in the Cameron Highlands, Malaysia, looking for something equally rootless—the rafflesia, the world's largest flower.

These flowers might be massive, but even so they are difficult to locate. They are rare and temperamental, only blooming for four to five days at a time. Sometimes there aren't any flowers for months. The plant's existence has also been threatened by a diminishing habitat, with sizable amounts of rainforest cleared for palm oil plantations or land development, which has made the rafflesia even scarcer.

As much as I love the adventure of a trek and finding things on my own, that's not an option in this situation. Because the rafflesia teeters on the verge of extinction and is considered a protected species, I have to hire a guide to venture anywhere near the flower. Also the rafflesia that grows in this part of Malaysia is found only on native land; only those in the Orang Asli tribe (or guides educated by the tribe) know where to find it.

My guide drives a navy blue Land Rover that looks like it has been dipped in caramel. Muddy caramel. Oozy mud coats the lower two-thirds of the vehicle, and I have no idea where this guy has been or where he's taking me, but I buckle up for a bumpy ride. He slides his slight frame into the driver's seat, and when he looks into the rearview mirror, I catch sight of his bulbous, bloodshot eyes. A silver marijuana leaf dangles on the chain around his neck. A laminated poem is posted above the steering wheel:

Stoners live and stoners die
Fuck the world, let's get high.
Pot's a plant, it grows in the ground,
If God didn't like it, it wouldn't be around.
So drink 151 and smoke a bowl,
Party hard and rock and roll.
To all you preps who think you're cool,
Fuck you, bitches. Stoners rule!

The man is a plant lover. That's all I'm saying.

Our drive is two hours on bone-jarring roads. At one point I am launched from my seat toward the ceiling, even though I'm wearing a seat belt, and I almost bruise myself on the roof.

Suddenly, at a remarkably unremarkable part of the road, the guide hits the brakes and turns off the ignition. Outside the vehicle, there are no paths and no signs, just a snarl of jungle. He motions for me to follow along.

The mud is ankle-deep, and the trek is a slog. We maneuver our bodies between trees, around prickly plants, through black and buzzy clouds of insects. We cross several bridges that don't look like bridges. They are nothing more than sticks of bamboo laid across ravines, with mud flowing fast and furious several feet below. One bridge in particular gives me pause, even though my guide has no problem crossing it. He seems annoyed when I hesitate.

"That's not a bridge," I say. "That's a big pair of chopsticks."

"It's bridge," he insists.

As I eye the chopsticks that are supposedly a bridge, a monkey scurries across it, and I swear he does a taunting dance at the end.

I reluctantly follow the primate's lead, though at a much slower place. But as I cautiously step forward, the sticks that form the bridge begin to roll, then fall away. The guide grasps my hand, pulling me up the slurpy side of the cliff just as I'm about to lose balance. Standing upright and looking back at the crumbled span, I have never felt more like Indiana Jones in my life.

We continue walking into the green vegetation, pushing leaves aside like heavy stage curtains. Sweat rolls down my back, and my loose tank top sticks to my skin.

"Shhh," the guide says. I don't know why he's whispering, but I am also quiet though I move with fervor. I am not a gardener or a woman who makes a hobby out of plants, but somehow finding this flower has become the most important thing to me at this moment in time. I need to see it. The guide halts, points his hand, and motions for me to gaze upon the majestic rafflesia bud.

It looks like a cabbage. A rotting cabbage. It's black but tinged with red, the color of goth nail polish, and it's the size of a bowling ball.

We move deeper into the jungle, again walking in silence, hiking a half mile before we see the bloom. It's substantial enough that it can be spotted from a distance, and it's vivid red. The color of my mom's favorite lipstick. It's also enormous, about as big around as a bistro table. My large feet look shrunken just standing next to it.

The petals are spongy, like a mushroom, with dots of fungus around the inside lip of the bloom. Inside, the central column is studded with projections, each the size of a pinkie finger but pointed like spikes.

This is a bizarre plant, with no leaves, no stems, no roots, not even any chlorophyll; technically it's an endoparasite that grows within vines. The flower is the only part that makes its way into the world and lives outside the host.

I blow gently on the bloom, and the scent that wafts back is a putrid mash-up of rotting hamburger and rotting fish. This is why the rafflesia is more commonly known as a corpse flower or corpse lily. (Not to be confused with the titan arum, an equally stinky plant that is called "corpse flower" for the same reason.)

I've had to cultivate a certain amount of faith to continue moving through the world. Along the way my grandmother died, immediately followed by the death of my mom, leaving me untethered, unmoored, aimless. I kept going because I knew there had to be something better ahead. I kept going because I didn't know how to turn back.

This flower before me, growing vibrantly and brilliantly in the midst of the jungle, seems to exist as a manifestation of that hope. It flourishes despite being rootless.

Sometimes I wonder what else I could have done for my mom. But what else was there to do? I couldn't have gone home to Ohio to wait bedside while she died. I am confident that those who are dying want their loved ones to live, which is exactly what my mom would have wanted for me. Why waste precious time suffering? And so I have carried her with me from Machu Picchu to the Great Pyramid to the convergence of seas. I chose life over her death.

And I will choose life again and again. I will spend the next week ambling over the tea plantations and floral hills of Malaysia. I will travel to South Korea, where I will eat plump kimchi dumplings in Seoul that pop sour and hot in my mouth and stay in chic, pulsing Hongdae, where music throbs all night long. I will travel past fences swathed in razor wire, landmines, and a river outfitted with metal spikes into the Demilitarized Zone that straddles North and South Korea. Stepping outside of the Joint Security Area, I will see North Korean tourists across the border; we aren't allowed to wave, but we will see each other. They'll take photos of me taking photos of them.

I will receive a summons for jury duty in California, and unable to postpone my civic duty, I will depart Korea with twenty-four dollars in my pocket and fly to Palm Springs. I will walk through the open-air Sonny Bono Concourse into the dry desert night to find my husband waiting with my dog, and they will both give me ecstatic kisses. A day later I will report to the courthouse, where I will be questioned and then dismissed by a judge who will have no idea what he's saying when he tells me, "You may go home."

Home will give me complicated spaces to travel. I won't have a job lined up, and my career path will not be clear. I'll have to get to know my husband all over again and figure out how to share a bed, a 600-square-foot apartment, and all of my choices with another person. Even simple acts will prove daunting. I will shop at stores that offer dozens of options for shampoos and cereals, and sometimes I will leave empty-handed rather than decide on just one.

Home will not be easy. But I purposely pushed myself into places of discomfort, emotionally, mentally, and physically, to change who I am at a fundamental level, and I cannot go back to the way things were. I don't want to. I have spent one year running down my grief, performing acts of love for my mom but also attempting to prove my own immortality.

In the midst of chasing life, I'll have discovered I am mortal, entirely and decidedly so, and that has to be enough. I will be fragile, I will be sorrowful, I will be wounded, and I will be capable of finding pinpricks of light among the darkness.

But before any of that, I am still standing in Malaysia, my skin coated with the brine of the jungle, my shoes caked with mud. The air is soggy, the land unruly, and I am here to appreciate the bold accomplishment of the rafflesia—how it grows tameless and untended, defying the odds. It doesn't burrow into the shadows; it finds a way out.

It shows me once again how regret must be risked in order to discover delight. Because the result is wilder, fiercer, and more exhilarating than you've imagined. And you? You are much braver than you think.

Epilogue

⤬⤬⤬

It is July 2018, and I am at Elephant Nature Park again. Only this time I'm not a volunteer; I'm a visitor. My husband stands behind me, and I'm holding the hand of a small, floppy-haired boy who is almost four.

Our son, Everest.

Jason and I gave him a name that conjures up a challenge, something powerful that stretches to the sky, a wish, a dream. It only seemed appropriate after miscarriage and difficulty conceiving in the first place. He came into our lives as a mighty hope.

This little left-handed boy loves broccoli and watermelon, dinosaurs, and David Bowie. He's a hiker, a dancer, a puzzle solver. Once, seeing a white piece of dandelion fluff float by on the breeze, he said, "Oh, look. A hummingbird ghost." He enjoys flopping facedown on top of a map and tracing roads with his pointer finger, asking the names of cities and far-flung places. He's also passionate about airplanes and wants to be a pilot. He says he will fly me to Greece.

We are traveling through Southeast Asia on a three-week vacation, and because Everest is already a laid-back, adaptable traveler, the twenty-hour flight from Los Angeles to Chiang Mai was a snap. We spent a few days walking the city, climbing temple stairs, and eating our way through night-market stalls. Now I have brought my family to a place that was significant on my solo travels.

I imagined this would be the closing of a loop, bringing my backpacking trip full circle. In all, my journey took me to seventeen countries over the course of one year. I achieved everything on my list for Mom—hiking the Inca Trail to Machu Picchu, trekking through the Amazon rainforest, volunteering at a monkey sanctuary, seeing the salt flats of Bolivia, attending a soccer game in Buenos Aires, going on safari in Kruger National Park, exploring the pyramids of Giza, visiting the ancient city of Petra, caring for elephants—and I accomplished many items on my own list. My travels also revealed how much I wanted to be a mother, something I didn't know about myself when I embarked on that journey.

Returning to Chiang Mai with my son is the culmination of everything meaningful in my life—my journey as a daughter and now as a mom—and I brace myself for an overwhelming, emotional moment. I assume Everest will take to the elephants right away, the way I did. He adores animal shows on TV, especially ones that feature elephants, and this is a rare opportunity to spend time with them up close.

But Everest doesn't care. He is shy around the elephants and visibly intimidated. I didn't think about what it must be like for him to see this creature in real life, outside the confines of a picture book or cartoon. They must appear 300 feet tall.

We stand on the wooden deck of a shelter as one of the rescued elephants lopes toward us and nudges her trunk toward my boy. I take half a watermelon and put it in Everest's hands. My son drops the melon, burrows into my side, and buries his face in my shirt.

"They're big," he murmurs.

I coach him through the process again, this time with a squash that is larger, thus easier for the elephant to grab without touching his hand. The elephant is gentle but playful. She taps her trunk on the squash and then swings the trunk toward herself again, as if to say, "For me?" Then she brings it back again and ever so gently plucks the squash from his palm. Everest doesn't notice. He's too busy looking up where a spider spins a web the size of a Volkswagen.

"Wow, Mom!" he cries out, excitedly. "Do you see that spider?"

I do. It's as big as his face.

"It's as big as my face!"

We spend an entire day with the elephants. We feed them, walk with them to the river to be bathed, watch them roam the stunning countryside. Elephant Nature Park has changed significantly in the seven years since I worked there, but only in positive ways. The sanctuary has expanded, and they've rescued more elephants. Stick Dog is no longer around, but there are hundreds of other rescue animals, both dogs and cats, and nice structures to house them. Also the efforts of my pothole-patching are long gone; the new road that leads to the park is smooth and well maintained. Eco-tourism has been embraced by Thailand, with dozens of other sanctuaries that have formed within the past several years; Elephant Nature Park paved the way.

Only one thing is missing: Mae Perm, the best friend and seeing-eye elephant for Jokia.

I spy Jokia from across a field, solitary under a thatched structure, and approach her gingerly. I can't say for a fact that Jokia remembers me. But it's a fact that I stand among a group of visitors, and Jokia reaches out to only one of us.

The air shifts. She tilts her head toward the sky, then stretches forward. She tucks the nub of her trunk in my hand, nuzzling me. It's said that elephants never forget, but research has shown that some elephants are even better with memories than others: matriarchs. The matriarchs of a herd develop strong social memories of their friends, their foes, their family members, because their survival depends on it.

A few tears roll down my cheeks, and Everest wipes them away.

"It's okay, Mom," he says. "Be happy."

I'm frustrated this trip doesn't hold as much meaning for Everest as I thought it would. At the same time, my own spirit shifts in unanticipated ways. I stand in between the gentle giant I fell for years ago and the gentle boy who claims my heart now, the hot Thai sun beaming down upon all of us. I never could have imagined this, my past and future colliding into one moment.

Elephants in the wild tend to travel the same paths, generation after generation, which might suggest memories don't die when one elephant does. The herd carries their memories forward.

I know Everest is young and that early experiences don't make much of an impression, but I say a silent prayer that this one will somehow stick. Maybe he will carry this memory forward long after I'm gone.

EVEREST WAS DOING THINGS IN HIS OWN TIME FROM THE start, coming into the world two weeks late during a C-section.

I've heard a lot of birth stories, and people always talk about the moment they saw their baby for the first time or felt the first touch of skin on skin. For me, I will always remember the brassy sound of my baby's first cry, slicing through the cold, white air of the operating room. Robbed of all my other senses—hands strapped down, nose clogged, a curtain blocking my view—that noise was how I first connected with my child, and it was golden, and it was perfect.

"It's a boy!" one of the doctors shouted. "Ten fingers, ten toes!" said another.

Someone brought the baby to my head and laid him next to my face. I nuzzled him with my cheek, and I felt like an animal—a cat rubbing her kitten—before he was swept away to a recovery room. He was wiped down, measured, swaddled, then returned to my chest.

When he settled upon my skin, I stared at him.

"Who are you?" I marveled. "Who are you going to be?"

The question ran through the days and months that followed, through long nights of nursing and diaper changes, through the moments when he peered back at me with enormous eyes, the black of his irises indistinguishable from his pupils. He was a colicky and unsettled baby, who pinched his face until he looked like a withered eggplant while he howled for hours. I cradled him tight and did my best to soothe the screams from his body, gingerly swaying back and forth in the yellow rocking chair where my mother once held me.

He grew quickly, part boy, part pony. As soon as he learned to climb out of his crib, he burst from his room each morning, spring-loaded with the energy of a colt emerging from a corral. He hardly crawled; he scaled the furniture and ran circles around the dinner table and somersaulted across the floor. Jason and I gave up on the baby gate after the first year of Everest's life, because it was rendered useless when he built ramps to hop over the top.

I will always wonder if I have condemned Everest to a life with Alzheimer's, either in his own body or caring for me if I have it in mine. But I have to have hope. That's the reason he's here, after all. Jason and I decided risk was a better path than regret.

In moments of doubt, I think back to experiencing the Badlands of South Dakota with my mom, both of us witnesses to the strange theatricality of the landscape, how ravaged it was and how magnificent. The world is too remarkable to keep to myself. I'm grateful to share it.

AFTER THAILAND, MY FAMILY HEADS TO CAMBODIA TO explore temples, visit Bill and Jill, and see the landmine clearing crew in action. We drive into the leafy countryside, a couple of hours away from Siem Reap, where a landmine has been found on a farm, not far from a path where children walk to school.

Everest dons the smallest protective vest, which is still enormous on his thirty-five-pound frame, and a helmet with a clear plastic face visor that goes all the way to his chest. After the team places dynamite around the old explosive, Everest presses the button to detonate it. We are close enough that he can see the plume of smoke above the treetops, hear the boom, and feel the earth shake, but he doesn't realize what happened until Bill carries him over to the farm where the landmine used to be, places him in the hole, and gives him a lollipop.

"You did this!" Bill says.

Then it's onward to Bali, a place none of us have traveled before.

Everest's last day of age three is spent by the ocean. I buy a pink cupcake from a bakery stand, and he eats it while playing in the sand, using his shoe to dig for treasure. And then I spy a treasure that wasn't on any of our maps: a small sea turtle conservation center in Sanur near the beach.

There are so many obstacles to a baby sea turtle's survival, which is why most sea turtle species around the world are endangered. The baby sea turtles hatch as a group, usually at night, and they dash toward the brightest horizon they can find. It used to be that moonlight led them to the ocean, but artificial light along the shore can be disorienting, outshining the natural light, and the hatchlings often head inland instead.

This is a problem because if the turtles don't make it to the ocean quickly, they can die of dehydration, from exposure to the elements, or at the claws of birds and crabs. Some turtles get caught in fishing nets near the beach or die from consuming litter. Many nesting sites are destroyed before the turtles ever have a chance to hatch.

Organizations like this one in Bali protect the turtle eggs and hatch them in a safe environment. When the hatchlings are old enough, volunteers release them into the ocean. And that's exactly what we do for Everest's birthday.

Thanks to TV programs, Everest knows words like "migration," "hibernation," and "camouflage," even if he hasn't seen the concepts presented in real life. We spend a little bit of time talking about the terms that might apply to the turtles. Then my son leans over a large tank where dozens of hatchlings swim.

"That one," he says. He points to a little turtle, smaller than a deck of cards, that appears to be bashing itself against the side of the tank and trying to climb out. In a tank full of frenetic baby turtles, my son has picked out the wildest one of all. Everest names him Spikey.

An employee from the organization fishes Spikey out of the water with a plastic bowl—you don't want to touch hatchlings with your hand—and then carefully gives the bowl to Everest. Step by gentle step we walk out of the center and out to the water.

At the ocean's edge, Everest pauses with a concerned look on his face. He asks how Spikey will know where to go.

"It's instinct, sweet pea."

"Instinct?"

"It means there's something in your body that tells you where to go, or what to do, or how to behave. It's like knowing without actually knowing you know," I say. "Instinct tells him that he must be out there, so he goes."

We wade out into the gentle waves, as deep as we can without Everest getting tugged away by the tide, and he lowers the bowl.

"Careful," Jason says, even though Everest is moving slowly, tenderly.

Spikey paddles from the shallow water that swirls around us and into the great expanse of the ocean. He swims past the fishing boats anchored nearby, past the bobbing buoys, and then into the vanishing point. That's where Spikey disappears from our view, traveling to places he doesn't know yet, traveling to places we someday might.

A warm breeze rustles my hair as I stand in the Bali Sea next to my husband and a boy on the precipice of his own adventures. We have no idea how far this journey will take us, only that we must embark on it.

Everest grabs my hand and whispers, "Go, Spikey, go."

ACKNOWLEDGMENTS

FIRST AND FOREMOST, I AM FOREVER GRATEFUL TO THE reader, the person who makes an effort to meet me on the page. I recognize that books are an investment of your time, energy, and sometimes money, and I'm thankful you made space in your life for my work.

I have so many people in my corner, it's not even a corner anymore; they've taken over the whole room. Thank you to my writing friends: my smart and inspiring hygges, Heather Scott Partington, Eileen Shields, and Lizi Gilad Silver; Mag Gabbert, who is a constant source of magic in my life; Leigh Raper, Kate Maruyama, Sara Marchant, John Mattson, all of whom listened to me groan about this book for years and offered gentle advice every time I was in a deep, dark hole; my MFA mentors and instructors; and everyone in my literary community, both online and off, especially the Binders.

I had a breakthrough at the Cambridge Writers' Workshop during a conversation with Alex Marzano-Lesnevich, which led to the chapter about the rafflesia flower and the ending I had been seeking. And when I was on a deadline, Steve De Jarnatt offered me a quiet place to write.

A trip like mine doesn't happen alone, and there were countless friends who championed my journey and contributed to it: they drove me to airports, sent me encouraging notes, connected me with other people. And then there were the generous friends I made all over the world: they opened their homes when I needed a place to stay, offered rides when I hitchhiked, fed me when I was hungry. I appreciate you all more than you'll ever know.

After my computer broke in Bolivia, then in Argentina, then again in South Africa, my friend Case Garrison crowdsourced the funds to buy me a reliable laptop, and that was before crowdsourcing was even a thing. I am thankful to everyone who chipped in; all my notes, my blog posts, my photos, and my early drafts of this book wouldn't have happened without you.

All my love to Karen Deitrick, who constantly demonstrates how to be a good friend. She drove all the way across the state of Ohio to spend time with me after my mom's funeral, and I don't have enough words to ever thank her.

Most of my relatives never understood why I needed to take this trip, but they humored me anyway and supported me the best way they knew how. A special shout-out goes to my cousin Tony, who has been my loudest and most enthusiastic fan, and my sister, who was my long-distance reading buddy while I traveled.

My dad still doesn't believe my book is going to be published, so if you've made it to this part, Dad, see! Though I'm sorry we had to walk the long, sorrowful road of Alzheimer's, I know grief strengthened our relationship. I love you.

Tod Goldberg, my friend–mentor–grad school director, helped give me the confidence to leave my newspaper job and aspire to be a better writer. He changed my life.

This book wouldn't be in your hands without Dan Smetanka, the editor who took a chance on me. He shared my vision from the start, and he pushed my writing to be stronger and fiercer. I'm grateful my book found such a good home at Counterpoint. Eternal thanks to Megan Fishmann for guiding this book toward an audience.

My agent Dara Hyde is the best possible representative I could ever ask for; she saw the best in me, even when I couldn't.

Of course I have to thank Jason, who knew the best way to love me was to let me go. He's my biggest cheerleader and the reason I came home again.

And Everest. My light, my life, the very best thing I've ever made with an egg. Someday you'll be old enough to read this, and I want you to know you're the reason I don't get much sleep. But you're also the reason I don't want to blink and risk missing a moment. I am thrilled I get to share this world with you.

This book is also for anyone who is a caregiver, who is a witness to a loved one's illness, or who is grieving. Though I can't take away your pain, I can sit with you in it. I wrote this book so you'd know you are not alone. The earth is big and kind and ready to embrace you.

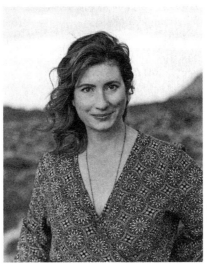

© Lance Gerber

MAGGIE DOWNS is an award-winning writer based in Palm Springs, California. Her work has appeared in *The New York Times*, *The Washington Post*, *Los Angeles Times*, *Palm Springs Life*, and *McSweeney's* and has been anthologized in *The Lonely Planet Travel Anthology: True Stories from the World's Best Writers* and *Best Women's Travel Writing*. *Braver Than You Think* is her first book. Find out more at maggiedowns.com.